WORKBOOK *to accompany*
Respiratory Care Pharmacology

D. Jones, RRT

D. Jones, PDT

WORKBOOK *to accompany*

Respiratory Care Pharmacology

CRYSTAL L. DUNLEVY, EdD, RRT

Visiting Professor
Department of Cardiopulmonary Care Sciences
Georgia State University
Atlanta, Georgia

FIFTH EDITION

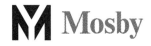 Mosby

St. Louis Baltimore Boston Carlsbad Chicago Minneapolis New York Philadelphia Portland
London Milan Sydney Tokyo Toronto

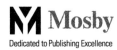

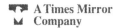

Publisher: Don E. Ladig
Editor: Janet Russell
Developmental Editor: Dina Shourd
Project Manager: Gayle Morris
Designer: Gail Hudson
Manufacturing Manager: Karen Lewis

Printed in the United States of America
Mosby, Inc.
11830 Westline Industrial Drive
St. Louis, Missouri 64146

International Standard Book Number: 0-8151-2004-4

98 99 00 01 02 / 9 8 7 6 5 4 3 2 1

Preface

The study of respiratory care pharmacology can be overwhelming, just by the very sound of the name. Committing to memory the chemical compositions, complicated interactions, and potential hazards of so many drugs is a daunting task. In writing the workbook to accompany *Respiratory Care Pharmacology, ed. 5*, by Joseph Rau, Jr., I've tried to always keep the students' perspective in mind. So that you can focus on the main ideas presented in the textbook and develop a thorough understanding of the basic concepts, I have included review discussions of main topics, as well as reinforcement of key points and definitions. Immediately following topic discussions, I have included quick review questions so that you can check your comprehension before moving on to the next section. You'll also be able to test your knowledge with clinical scenarios and practice board questions. Answers to all of the questions are listed in an appendix at the back of the book. Included at no extra cost is a light-hearted approach to learning that I have found to be successful in teaching any subject—the text is written pretty much the way I talk.

I sincerely hope that this workbook will make an important, but intimidating, subject a little easier to absorb. If you happen to have some fun along the way, thank my former students!

To Blair, Cole, and Bill for really writing this book but allowing me to take the credit. I know it's corny to thank your parents, but thanks, Mom and Dad.

Crystal L. Dunlevy, EdD, RRT

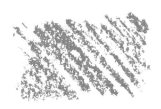

Table of Contents

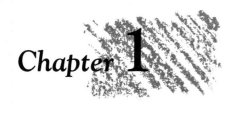

Chapter 1 Introduction to Respiratory Care Pharmacology

Before you delve into a text on respiratory care pharmacology, you should be familiar with a few basic definitions.

Pharmacology Definitions

1. Drug—any chemical that changes an organism's function
2. Pharmacology—the study of drugs (chemicals)
3. Respiratory care pharmacology—applying pharmacology to the treatment of cardiopulmonary disease and critical care
4. Therapeutics—treating disease with drugs
5. Toxicology—the study of poisonous substances and their pharmacological actions

*Q*1. Respiratory care pharmacology applies the study of _____ to the treatment of _____ and _____.

*Q*2. If Dr. Jekyll were to work on discovering an antidote for the secret formula that turned him into Mr. Hyde, he would be engaged in _____.

Naming Drugs

By the time a drug gets official approval for use in the United States, it will have been given at least five different names:

1. Chemical name—name that indicates the drug's chemical structure

2. Code name—name (like RT#007!) given to an experimental chemical that shows promise as a drug
3. Generic name—the non-proprietary name (Example: ibuprofen; acetaminophen)
4. Official name—what the generic name becomes once it gets official approval (the examples above are also official names)
5. Trade name—brand name; proprietary name given to a drug by the manufacturer (Example: Trade names for ibuprofen include Advil and Motrin; Tylenol is a trade name for acetaminophen.)

*Q*3. Which two names above can be identical?
   a. Code and chemical
   b. Chemical and generic
   c. Generic and official
   d. Official and trade

*Q*4. Which name is equivalent to the brand name?
   a. Code
   b. Generic
   c. Official
   d. Trade

Sources of Drug Information

If you want to get information about a drug, there are several places you can look. The "official" source of info about drug standards is the *United States Pharmacopeia–National Formulary (USP-NF)*. This gets revised continuously, so it's a good source. It's published by the American Pharmaceutical Association.

The *Physician's Desk Reference*, commonly known as the *PDR*, is put together by drug manufacturers (this may make it less objective than the *USP-NF*). This has lots of color charts that identify drugs, lists manufacturers, and tells how the drugs work, when they're indicated and contraindicated, and possible side effects.

Another place to look is the American Society of Hospital Pharmacists' the *Hospital Formulary*. This book gives more general info about classes of drugs (like antibiotics and antidepressants)

*Q*5. Which is the most objective source of information about specific drugs?
   a. *USP-NF*
   b. *PDR*
   c. *Hospital Formulary*

Sources of Drugs

Most of today's drugs come from chemicals, but plants, minerals, and animals also contain certain active ingredients for drugs.

For hundreds of years, Native, South, and Central Americans and the Chinese have used plants, minerals, and animals for their active ingredients in the treatment of heart disease and asthma and as poison (*Dr. Quinn, Medicine Woman* does it all the time!) Poppy seeds are well known for containing opium. (No wonder Dorothy and Toto got sleepy.) Check out the text for more examples.

Process of Drug Approval in the United States

It's really time consuming and expensive to get a drug approved in the United States. To make it worse, most chemicals that were identified as potential drugs (remember RT#007?) don't ever make it to the general clinical use stage. Here's how it's done:

1. Chemical Identification—A chemical is identified that shows potential for having some useful physiologic effect. Researchers figure out the exact chemical structure and characteristics of the active ingredient during this phase.

2. Animal Studies—Animal studies are done so that the general effect of the drug, as well as its effect on specific organs, can be determined before human subjects are involved. Toxicology studies are also done during this phase (like determining how much of the chemical it takes to cause cancer and how fertility is affected).

3. Investigational New Drug (IND) Approval—Next, an IND application outlining plans for human studies has to be submitted to the FDA. Human studies are done in three phases and take about 3 years to finish.

   • Phase 1—includes a small number of healthy subjects
   • Phase 2—includes a small number of people who have the disease that the drug will treat
   • Phase 3—includes a large number of people with the disease at different centers around the country

4. New Drug Application (NDA)—Once the IND process is over (and successful), an NDA gets filed with the Food and Drug Administration (FDA). If it gets final approval, the drug is released for clinical use. Hooray! Detailed reports about every aspect of the drug and its use are in place for 6 months.

$\mathcal{Q}$6. Put the steps of the drug approval process in order from 1 to 4.

_____ animal studies

_____ NDA

_____ chemical identification

_____ IND

Food and Drug Administration New Drug Classification System

New drugs are classified by the FDA with a number followed by a hyphen and a letter, as follows:

A. important therapeutic gain over other drugs

AA. important therapeutic gain; for patients with acquired immunodeficiency syndrome (AIDS); fast track

B. modest therapeutic gain

C. little or no therapeutic gain

_____ 1. new chemical

_____ 2. new salt form

_____ 3. new dosage form

_____ 4. new combination

_____ 5. generic drug

_____ 6. new indication

Orphan Drugs

An orphan drug is one that is used to diagnose or treat a rare disease (affecting fewer than 200,000 people). These drugs may also be used to treat a disease that's not so rare (affecting more than 200,000 people), but the development and marketing of the drug are not cost effective. In other words, the amount of money that it costs to develop and market the drug is a lot more than the money that the manufacturer takes in through sales. Check out the text for examples of orphan drugs.

$\mathcal{Q}$7. List one advantage and one disadvantage of orphan drugs.

Advantage: _____

_____

_____

Disadvantage: _____

_____

_____

The Prescription

The prescription is the written order for a drug. It contains instructions for the pharmacist and the patient about how to make, dispense, and take the drug.

To prescribe narcotics or controlled substances, a physician must have a Drug Enforcement Administration (DEA) registration number.

Here are the parts of a prescription:

1. Patient's name, address, and the date
2. Rx—meaning recipe; this is the *superscription*
3. *Inscription*—name of drug and the amount prescribed
4. *Subscription*—direction to the pharmacist about preparation
5. "Sig"—directions to the patient (some medications must be taken on an empty stomach, some with milk; how many tablets, how many times a day, etc.)
6. Prescriber's name—the physician's name

Indicate whether the following statements are true or false.

_____ $\mathcal{Q}$8. The sig part of a prescription contains the physician's signature.

_____ $\mathcal{Q}$9. The subscription contains the name and amount of drug prescribed.

Over-the-Counter Drugs

Over-the-counter (OTC) drugs are drugs that anyone can buy without a prescription. Anything on the drugstore shelf is considered OTC. Examples include cough syrups, aspirin, and hydrocortisone creams. The most common respiratory example is Primatene Mist—it's epinephrine that can be bought OTC.

Inappropriate use of OTC respiratory drugs can cause death because people medicate themselves and don't go to the emergency department or their physician until their asthma is out of control.

Q 10. List three examples of OTC drugs.
1. _____
2. _____
3. _____

Generic Substitution in Prescriptions

Generic substitution is designed to save the patient money. The physician has to write on the prescription that it's okay to use the generic form of the drug. Generic forms of OTC drugs are also less expensive—like the Kroger brand of ibuprofen versus Advil.

Respiratory Care Pharmacology Overview

Aerosolized Agents Given by Inhalation

Aerosolized agents given by inhalation represent a common group of drugs used in respiratory care. The aerosol route provides local topical treatment to the upper and lower airway.

The oral and nasal routes of inhalation have five advantages over other routes of drug administration (like intravenous or intramuscular):

1. Smaller doses may be given because the drug is acting directly on the airway.
2. Side effects are usually fewer and less severe (partly because of the smaller dose).
3. Onset of action is quick.
4. Delivery of the drug is targeted to the respiratory system.
5. Inhalation of aerosol drugs is painless, safe, and convenient.

A great summary of the different classes of aerosol drugs, their uses, and their generic names is listed in the text.

Q 11. Match the class of aerosol drug with its generic name.
   a. pentamidine
   b. acetylcysteine
   c. albuterol
   d. cromolyn sodium
   e. beractant
   f. dexamethasone
   g. ipratropium bromide

_____ 1. anticholinergic agents
_____ 2. antiasthmatic agents
_____ 3. exogenous surfactants
_____ 4. corticosteroids
_____ 5. adrenergic agents
_____ 6. mucoactive agents
_____ 7. antiinfective agents

Related Drug Groups in Respiratory Care

The following drug groups are also important because they're often used in critical care:

1. Antiinfective agents—drugs used to treat infections, like antibiotics and antifungal drugs
2. Neuromuscular blocking agents—these paralyze people and are used in critical care because paralyzed patients need to have their ventilation supported (their diaphragm is also paralyzed) (Example: curare)

Aerosolized agents

Drug group	Therapeutic purpose	Agents
Adrenergic agents	Beta-adrenergic: Relaxation of bronchial smooth muscles and bronchodilation, to reduce R_{aw} and improve ventilatory flow rates in airway obstruction such as COPD, asthma, CF, acute bronchitis Alpha-adrenergic: Epinephrine—topical vasoconstriction and decongestion	Epinephrine Isoproterenol Isoetharine Terbutaline Metaproterenol Albuterol Pirbuterol Bitolterol Salmeterol
Anticholinergic agents	Relaxation of cholinergic-induced bronchoconstriction to improve ventilatory flow rates in COPD and asthma	Ipratropium bromide
Mucoactive agents	Modification of the properties of respiratory tract mucus; current agents lower viscosity and promote clearance of secretions	Acetylcysteine Dornase alfa
Corticosteroids	Reduce and control the inflammatory response in the airway usually associated with asthma (lower respiratory tract) or with seasonal or chronic rhinitis (upper respiratory tract)	Dexamethasone Beclomethasone dipropionate Triamcinolone acetonide Flunisolide Fluticasone propionate Budesonide
Antiasthmatic agents	To prevent the onset and development of the asthmatic response, through inhibition of chemical mediators of inflammation	Cromolyn sodium Nedocromil sodium Zafirlukast Zileuton
Antiinfective agents	To inhibit or eradicate specific infective agents, such as *Pneumocystis carinii* (pentamidine) or respiratory syncytial virus (ribavirin)	Pentamidine Ribavirin
Exogenous surfactants	Approved clinical dose is by direct intratracheal instillation, for the purpose of restoring a more normal lung compliance in respiratory distress syndrome of the newborn	Colfosceril palmitate Beractant

CF, Cystic fibrosis; *COPD*, chronic obstructive pulmonary disease.

3. Central nervous system agents—analgesics (pain killers), sedatives, and hypnotics (Example: morphine)

4. Antiarrhythmic agents—drugs that treat dangerous cardiac dysrhythmias (Example: lidocaine)

5. Antihypertensive and antianginal agents—drugs to treat high blood pressure and chest pain (Example: beta blockers; nitroglycerin)

6. Anticoagulants and thrombolytic agents—drugs to keep blood from clotting (Example: heparin)

7. Diuretics—used when patients need to get rid of excess body fluid (whether it's in the lungs, heart, etc.) (Example: furosemide)

𝒬 12. Antibiotics are classified as _____ _____.

𝒬 13. Drugs that control or prevent cardiac dysrhythmias are classified as _____ _____.

Now that you've had a chance to review this material from the text, try the five questions that follow. The references at the end of each question tell you where to look in the text if you're having trouble answering the question. When you're finished, check your responses with the answer key at the end of the book.

1. Animal studies are designed to accomplish which of the following?
   a. General effect on the organism
   b. Effects on specific organs
   c. Toxicology studies
   d. all the above   (Chapter 1, p. 6)

2. Studies involving human subjects occur during which stage of the drug approval process?
   a. Chemical identification
   b. IND approval
   c. NDA
   d. Internal review   (Chapter 1, p. 6)

3. How many phases of study must be successfully completed on a new drug before it is granted FDA approval?
   a. One
   b. Two
   c. Three
   d. Four   (Chapter 1, p. 6)

4. The FDA has classified a new drug as 6-B. What does this mean?
   a. New chemical; indicated for patients with AIDS
   b. New indication; modest therapeutic gain
   c. Generic drug; little therapeutic gain
   d. New chemical; important therapeutic gain   (Chapter 1, p. 7)

5. Which of the following is an advantage of the oral route of aerosol drug delivery?
   a. Fewer side effects
   b. Slow onset of action
   c. Larger doses are required
   d. All are advantages
            (Chapter 1, p. 9)

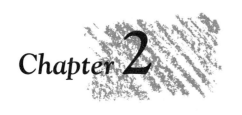

Chapter 2   Principles of Drug Action

To understand how a drug works from the time it's given to the time it takes effect, you need to understand the three phases that it progresses through. These stages areas follow:

Pharmaceutical Phase—how the drug is made available to the body

Pharmacokinetic Phase—how the drug gets absorbed, distributed, metabolized, and eliminated

Pharmacodynamic Phase—how the drug causes an effect in the body

Pharmaceutical Phase

Definition: the method by which a drug dose is made available to the body. Basically, this depends on how the drug is available (pill, cream, etc.) and how it's given (injection, inhalation, etc.). Let's start with the dosage forms.

Drug Dosage Forms

How the drug is physically available must be compatible with how you're going to give it. Many drugs are available in more than one form. For example, if you're stressed over a pharmacology exam and need Pepto-Bismol, you'll be forced to take it orally—you can't inhale it!

Table 2-1 lists common formulations for different routes of administration.

Indicate whether the following statement is true or false.

_____ *Q*1. Almost all drugs are only available in one form.

Drug formulations and additives

Even though the drug is the active ingredient in a formulation, it's probably not the only ingredient. Some capsules are made of gelatinous material along with the drug, so that you can easily swallow it. Aerosolized forms of drugs usually have propellants (metered dose inhalers—MDIs), preservatives, and/or carrier agents (dry powder inhalers—DPIs).

Routes of Administration

Oral route—You've got to be able to swallow to take medication this way. The oral route is used frequently because it's safe, convenient, and painless (unlike the injection route). On the other hand, medication delivered this way doesn't take effect as quickly as it does if you use parenteral administration. To take a drug by the

Table 2-1   Three different dosage forms for the bronchodilator drug, albuterol, indicating ingredients other than active drug

	Nebulizer solution	Metered dose inhaler	Dry powder inhaler
ACTIVE DRUG: INGREDIENTS:	Albuterol sulfate Benzalkonium chloride, sulfuric acid	Albuterol Trichloromonofluoromethane, dichlorodifluoromethane, oleic acid	Albuterol Lactose

oral route, the patient must have intact airway protective reflexes, so the patient doesn't aspirate it. If the drug makes it through the stomach and gets absorbed into the blood stream, a *systemic effect* is what you get.

Injectable (parenteral) route—If you want to split hairs, *parenteral* means *any route of administration other than oral.* However, the term usually means *injection* when it's used in the clinical setting (or on *General Hospital*). When a drug is injected, a local or a systemic effect can be produced. For example, intravenous (IV) administration of lidocaine produces a systemic effect, but if you inject lidocaine subcutaneously, the effect is local anesthetic. There are four ways to inject a drug:

- Subcutaneous (sc)—injected into the subcutaneous tissue (hence, the name), beneath both the epidermis and the dermis
- Intramuscular (IM)—injected into the muscle layer, deeper than sc (ouch!)
- Intravenous (IV)—injected into the vein
- Intrathecal—injected into the spinal canal

Topical route—Drugs can be applied to the skin or mucous membranes, to produce a local or systemic effect. An example of a drug applied to the skin for a local effect is hydrocortisone cream for hives. An example of a drug applied to the skin for a systemic effect is the nicotine patch.

Inhalation route—You can also get a local or a systemic effect by inhaling a drug. If you inhale a bronchodilator, it will exert a local effect on the airways. If you inhale nitrous oxide (used clinically for anesthesia), you will get a systemic effect. Local delivery of a drug is associated with fewer side effects.

Place a check under the effect that you get with each of the following routes of administration:

	LOCAL	SYSTEMIC	EITHER
Q2. Topical	___	___	___
Q3. Oral	___	___	___
Q4. Inhalation	___	___	___
Q5. Injection	___	___	___

Pharmacokinetic Phase

Definition: the time course and deposition of a drug in the body, based on its absorption, distribution, metabolism, and elimination.

Absorption

For a drug to work, it's got to be absorbed. There are four ways for a drug to be absorbed:

1. Aqueous diffusion—Aqueous diffusion occurs in aqueous compartments of the body, like interstitial spaces or inside a cell. The drug diffuses across the cell membrane by a concentration gradient.

2. Lipid diffusion—For a drug to be distributed in the body, it's got to cross a lot of epithelial membranes before it gets to the target organ. Epithelial cells have lipid membranes, so for the drug to get across, it's got to be lipid soluble. Nonionized drugs are lipid soluble; ionized forms of drug are water soluble (lipid insoluble). Nonionized molecules are well absorbed into the blood stream and across the blood-brain barrier. Lipid diffusion is passive.

3. Facilitated transport—In some cases special carrier molecules can carry substances across membranes. Facilitated diffusion requires energy.

4. Endocytosis/exocytosis—In endocytosis a cell membrane surrounds a substance and absorbs it into the inside of the cell, where that substance is released. Exocytosis is just the opposite—the cell releases a substance from inside, instead of absorbing it.

Q6. Which drug/type is best absorbed into the blood stream? Circle as many as are correct.

nonionized   ionized
lipid-soluble   water-soluble

*Q*7. Explain in your own words the difference between aqueous diffusion and facilitated transport. _____

(It should only take a few words. That's why there's not much space!)

Distribution

To be effective, a drug has to have a certain concentration. This concentration is determined partly by the rate of absorption versus the rate of elimination and partly by the volume of drug. A drug will be distributed to one or more body compartments. These compartments and their corresponding volumes are listed in Table 2-2.

Table 2-2 Volumes (approximate) of major body compartments

Compartment	Volume (L)
Vascular (blood)	5
Interstitial fluid	10
Intracellular fluid	20
Fat (adipose tissue)	14–25

$$\frac{\text{Volume of}}{\text{Distribution (VD)}} = \frac{\text{Drug amount/}}{\text{Concentration of drug}}$$

You can get the drug concentration from a blood sample. But because the drug may be distributed in a compartment other than the vascular one, the calculated volume of distribution can be larger than the blood volume. For this reason, volume of distribution is referred to as the *apparent volume of distribution (AVD)*.

You can use VD to determine an appropriate dose for a given therapeutic level, if you rearrange the equation.

Example: To get a theophylline concentration of 10 mg/L, with a VD of 35 L, what dose do you give?

$$VD = \text{amount/concentration}$$
$$\text{Amount (dose)} = VD \times \text{concentration}$$
$$\text{Dose} = 35\,L \times 10\,\text{mg/L} = 350\,\text{mg}$$

*Q*8. See how easy it is! Now you try. What's the AVD (in liters) if I give a 100-mg dose of a drug whose concentration is 5 mg/L? _____

Metabolism

The liver is the main (but not the only) site of drug metabolism. The lung and the intestinal wall can metabolize drugs too. The liver contains enzymes that convert lipid-soluble molecules into water-soluble *metabolites,* which are more easily excreted. Chronic abuse or administration of a drug that is metabolized by the enzymes in the liver can cause these enzyme levels to increase. This is called *enzyme induction.* This may affect the dose required to produce a therapeutic effect. Patients with chronic obstructive pulmonary disease(COPD) are often prescribed theophylline. If they smoke cigarettes, the breakdown of theophylline is increased, so they may have to take a higher dose to get a therapeutic effect. This is a *bad* thing!

Another clinical piece of info that you should know is called the *first-pass effect.* If you take a drug orally, and it gets absorbed into the blood from the stomach, the portal vein will drain this blood directly into the liver. The blood from the liver drains into the right and left hepatic veins, into the inferior vena cava, and into the general circulation. If the liver enzymes metabolize the drug, most of the drug's effect will be lost in passing into the liver, before it even gets to the general circulation. This is the *first-pass effect.* The other routes of administration avoid this nasty business because they drain into the venous circulation so that the drugs slosh around (are distributed) in the body for a while before they even get to the liver, where they are metabolized!

Certain genetic differences among people can influence the rate at which a drug is metabolized.

In the following sentence, circle the one correct answer.

*Q*9. The first-pass effect (increases, decreases, doesn't affect) the amount of drug that's available to exert a systemic effect.

Elimination

The main site of drug elimination is the kidney. *Drug clearance* is the ratio of rate of elimination to concentration of a drug in body fluid. The *rate of elimination* is the amount of drug eliminated from the body per hour. The *half-life* of a drug is the amount of time it takes to reduce the amount of drug in the body by one half during elimination. A drug's half-life is very important for determining the frequency of dosing. If you dose faster than the half-life time, drug accumulation and toxicity may result. This may result in nasty side effects and/or death. To achieve a steady drug level in the body, dosing must equal elimination.

The concentration of a drug in the body over time can be graphed as a time-plasma curve. The curve's shape describes a *bioavailability profile*, which can tell you whether the dose you've given is enough to produce a therapeutic effect. Following are examples. Let's pretend they're bronchodilators.

The short-acting curve (A) might represent a drug like isoetharine that reaches peak effect quickly and doesn't last long. Although such a drug wouldn't be great for maintenance therapy, it would do the job during an asthma attack. The intermediate curve (B) might be albuterol, with 30- to 60-minute peak effect and 4- to 6-hour duration. Albuterol would be good for maintenance therapy if you took it, but it probably wouldn't last you through the night. Curve C might be salmeterol. This would last a long time (up to 12 hours) but not peak for 1 to 2 hours, so it would only be good for maintenance.

*Q*10. BD has asthma. Which bronchodilator should she take for maintenance therapy?
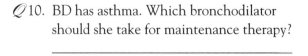

*Q*11. Why?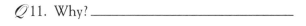

*Q*12. Which should she take during an asthma attack?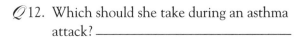

*Q*13. Why?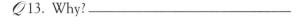

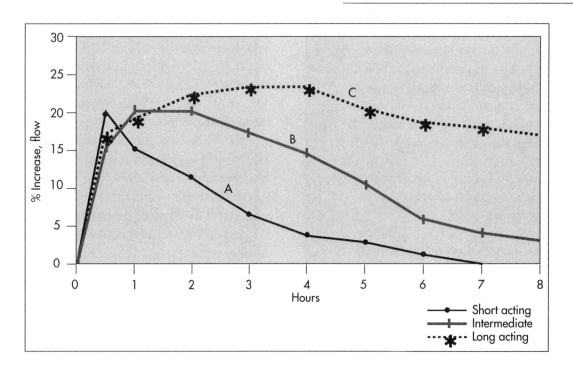

Pharmacokinetics of Inhaled Aerosols

Local Versus Systemic Effect

Inhaled aerosols are deposited on the surfaces of the upper and lower airways, so they're really topically administered. Remember, topical administration can cause a local or systemic effect.

An example of a local effect would be nasal inhalation of a vasoconstrictor, like oxymetazoline (Afrin), or inhalation of a bronchodilator to dilate the lower airways. An example of a systemic effect through inhalation is the experimental administration of insulin through the nose for systemic control of diabetes.

Inhaled aerosols used to treat pulmonary diseases are intended to have a local effect on the lung and airways, delivering maximal deposition in the lung with minimal systemic side effects.

Because a certain percentage of the aerosol that you deliver by inhalation is swallowed, gastrointestinal absorption occurs right along with lung absorption. Guess which one is higher? Ninety percent of aerosolized drug is swallowed! Can you believe it?! Only about 10% gets to the airways, like it's supposed to.

Q 14. Think inhaled aerosol. List one advantage of a local versus a systemic effect when administering a drug this way.

_____

_____

Swallowed Aerosol

One of two things can happen to the aerosolized drug that gets swallowed:

1. It can be absorbed from the stomach and metabolized in a first-pass effect through the liver.

2. It can be inactivated in the intestinal wall as it's absorbed into the portal circulation.

Generally, if the first-pass metabolism is high, systemic drug levels will be low (because the drug is getting flushed out faster). If first-pass metabolism is low (more of the drug is swallowed), systemic drug levels will be higher and may cause side effects.

Q 15. How much of an inhaled aerosol gets swallowed? _____

Q 16. How much of it gets to your lungs? _____

_____

Inhaled Aerosol

Aerosol drugs supposedly interact with all the stuff in the airway—secretions, smooth muscle, nerve endings, etc. The drug may be absorbed into the bronchial circulation, which drains into the atria of the heart, and then goes out into systemic circulation. Nobody knows exactly how aerosolized drugs, like bronchodilators, get to the right receptors, so there's nothing to learn here! Okay—break's over.

Lung Availability/Total Systemic Availability Ratio

Lung availability/total systemic availability (L/T) basically tells how efficient aerosol delivery to the lung is. L/T ratio is defined as the proportion of drug available from the lung, out of the total amount systemically available.

As you've learned, the therapeutic effect of a bronchodilator depends on the amount of drug deposited on the airways; the side effects depend on the amount of drug absorbed into the system. L/T ratio gives you an idea of desired local effect in relation to unwanted systemic effect. If an inhalation device was perfectly efficient, all the drug would go to the lung and none would be available for gastrointestinal absorption. The L/T would be 1 (Lung availability = Total systemic availability). L/T ratio won't tell you whether side effects or toxicity will occur, though.

𝒬17. Which L/T ratio represents the most efficient aerosol delivery? Circle one.

1:2   1:3   1:4   1:5

Pharmacodynamic Phase

Definition: the mechanism of drug action (how it works)—the way the drug causes its effect on the body.

For a drug to cause any effect in the body, it has to combine with a *receptor*.

Structure-Activitiy Relation

The drug and the receptor must be structurally similar for matching to occur. The structure-activity relation (SAR) describes the relationship between the chemical structure of the drug and its clinical effect. Take isoproterenol and albuterol as examples. They have similar chemical structures, so they will both match to airway receptors. But the chemical structures are different enough to make a clinical difference—isoproterenol will also match with receptors found in the heart, which may cause increased heart rate in patients who receive this drug. Albuterol has a longer side chain (part of its chemical structure), which makes it more selective, so that it only matches with receptors in the airways. It's sort of like those old skeleton keys they used on TV to lock jail cells in the Old West—the key was pretty simple, so it could unlock more than just one door. But the key to your Volvo has so many nicks and notches in it that it will only unlock your car, and not the BMW parked next to you.

𝒬18. Circle one. The more complex the chemical structure of a drug, the (more, fewer) receptors it will match.

Nature and Type of Drug Receptors

Most drug receptors are proteins whose shape and electrical charge make them a match for a drug's shape and charge. For this "matching" to

occur, a process called *transmembrane signaling* has to occur. This can happen in one of four different ways.

1. Lipid-soluble drugs cross the cell membrane and act on receptors in the cell to initiate a drug response. Corticosteroids work this way.

𝒬19. Flashback. Are lipid-soluble drugs ionized or nonionized? _____

2. The drug attaches to the extracellular part of the receptor, projects into the cytoplasm, and starts an enzyme system that produces the desired effect. Insulin is an example of this process.

3. The drug attaches to a receptor on the surface of the membrane, which opens an ion channel for the drug to move through. Acetylcholine receptors on skeletal muscle work this way.

4. The drug attaches to a transmembrane receptor that is hooked up to an intracellular membrane by something called a G protein. Beta-adrenergic agents work via this process. There is a G protein (Gs) that stimulates an enzyme called adenylyl cyclase. This causes bronchodilation. Another G protein (Gi) inhibits adenylyl cyclase, which has the opposite effect on bronchial smooth muscle.

𝒬20. An increase in _____ protein stimulates _____, causing bronchodilation. This is an example of _____.

Dose-Response Relations

The body's response to a drug is directly proportional to the drug's concentration. As more drug is given, more receptors are occupied, so drug effect will increase up to the point where all receptor sites are occupied. The dose where 50% of the maximal response occurs is called effective dose (ED50). This refers to a drug's *potency*.

The *maximal effect* of a drug is the greatest response that can be produced by the drug so that even at a higher dose, you won't get any more response.

The more potent a drug is, the less it takes to produce 50% of the maximal response. For example, if drug A can elicit 50% maximal response with 2 mg, but it takes 4 mg of drug B to do the same thing, drug A is twice as potent as drug B.

Two drugs might have the same potency but different maximal effects. Check out the dose-response curves below:

Even though these two drugs have the same potency (ED50), drug B has a greater maximal effect than drug C.

Therapeutic index (TI) is also based on the dose-response curve of a drug. The difference here is, you're looking for an all-or-nothing response from subjects—they either improve or they don't. Improvement is quantified using ED50—the dose where half of the test subjects improve. On the flip side, lethal dose (LD50) represents the dose that will be lethal to 50% of the population of test subjects. Eek—needless to say, animals are used for the test population! Now for the definition you've been waiting for:

$$TI = ED50/LD50$$

TI gives you an idea of how safe the drug is. The smaller the TI, the more dangerous the drug (ED50 and LD50 are closer, so don't screw up your patient's prescription!). For example, penicillin has a high TI (around 100)—lethal and effective doses are really far apart, so it's a safe drug. Digitalis, on the other hand, has a TI of about 1.5, so be careful.

Q 21. Which drug is more potent? drug A (ED50 = 10 mg) or drug B (ED50 = 6 mg)?

Q 22. TI of a drug is 3. This drug is relatively (safe, dangerous).

Agonists and Antagonists

An *agonist* is a drug that binds to a receptor (affinity) and causes a response (efficacy)—it's got affinity plus efficacy. A full agonist gives you a greater maximal response than a partial agonist—duh!

Q 23. Does this mean that a partial agonist has less affinity or less efficacy?

_____

An *antagonist* can bind to the receptor but doesn't cause a response—it's got affinity but no efficacy. Worse yet, an antagonist can hog the receptor site and keep other drugs from reaching the receptor site. Very rude.

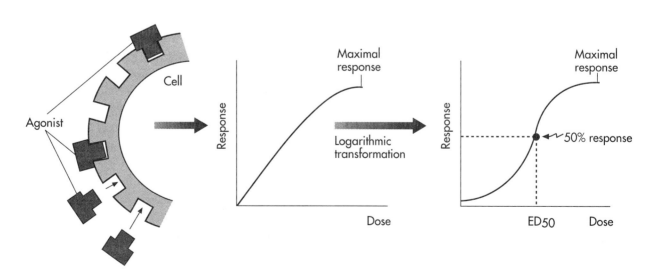

Q24. Affinity + Efficacy = _____

Q25. Affinity − Efficacy = _____

Positive interactions between drugs fall into three categories:

1. Synergism (1 + 1 = 3)—the effect of two drugs is greater than the sum of the effect of each drug alone.

2. Additive (1 + 1 = 2)—the maximal effect of two drugs is the sum of the effect of each drug alone

3. Potentiation (0 + 1 = 2)—In this type of synergism one drug doesn't produce any effect by itself, but if you give it with another drug, it will increase that drug's effect.

The following four terms describe an individual's response to a drug:

1. Idiosyncratic—like your wacky uncle—the drug has the opposite effect, an unusual effect, or no effect compared to the effect it's supposed to have.

2. Hypersensitivity—an allergic or immune-related response to a drug that can be quite serious, even requiring ventilatory support

3. Tolerance—less response to a drug over time—requires more of the drug to produce the same effect

4. Tachyphylaxis—rapid decrease in responsiveness to a drug

Match the following drug interactions with their mathematical definition:

Additive	1 + 0 = 2
Potentiation	1 + 1 = 3
Synergism	1 + 1 = 2

Q26. Diphenhydramine (Benadryl) makes most people drowsy, but it makes me hyper. This is an example of _____ _____ response.

And now, the moment you've been waiting for—10 NBRC-type questions! All the references at the end are from the text.

1. Which phase of drug action describes dose forms?
   a. Pharmaceutical
   b. Pharmacokinetic
   c. Pharmacodynamic
   d. Pharmacongaline   (Chapter 2, p. 12)

2. Which of the following is the only route of administration that cannot exert a local effect?
   a. Topical
   b. Oral
   c. Parenteral
   d. Inhalation   Chapter 2, p. 13)

3. Which type of drugs crosses the blood-brain barrier most easily?
   I.   nonionized
   II. ionized
   III. lipid-soluble
   IV. water-soluble

   a. I and III
   b. I and IV
   c. II and III
   d. II and IV   (Chapter 2, p. 14)

4. Which of the following is the main site of drug metabolism?
   a. Kidney
   b. Stomach
   c. Lung
   d. Liver   (Chapter 2, p. 17)

5. Which of the following is the main site of drug elimination?
   a. Intestine
   b. Stomach
   c. Kidney
   d. Liver   (Chapter 2, p. 19)

6. If a drug is administered more frequently than the half-life of the drug, which of the following may result?
   a. Synergy
   b. Accumulation
   c. Elimination
   d. Clearance   (Chapter 2, p. 19)

7. Which of the following time-plasma curves would be desirable for a drug designed for maintenance of a disease (including overnight)?
   Place examples from Figure 2-5 here in the following order...A—B—C—flat line
   a. B
   b. C
   c. A
   d. Flat line   (Chapter 2, p. 20)

8. Inhaled aerosols used in the treatment of pulmonary disease are intended to exert what effect on the lung?
   a. Local
   b. Systemic
   c. Kinetic
   d. Dynamic   (Chapter 2, p. 21)

9. The drug dose where 50% of its maximal response occurs is termed ED50. This refers to what aspect of the drug?
   a. Maximal effect
   b. Half-life
   c. Potency
   d. Bioavailability   (Chapter 2, p. 30)

10. Which of the following terms is used to describe what happens when an individual experiences less response to a drug over time?
    a. Hypersensitivity
    b. Idiosyncratic
    c. Toxicity
    d. Tolerance   (Chapter 2, p. 32)

Sim

RE is a 14-year-old boy who has been brought to the emergency room by his dad after having a high fever with shaking chills for the past 24 hours. RE states that he has had bronchitis for the past couple of weeks that he can't seem to shake. He says that he is short of breath; his respiratory rate is 32 breaths/min; his heart rate is 108; and he looks a little dusky. Auscultation reveals bilateral crackles in the lower lobes, with slight wheezing on inspiration. After examining him, both you and the physician agree that RE probably has pneumonia. RE will need a bronchodilator for the wheezing and antibiotics for the pneumonia. Which route(s) of administration would be best to deliver them?

_____
_____
_____
_____
_____

Answer: The oral or the parenteral routes are likely choices to give the antibiotics. Because RE's pneumonia seems to be advanced, the parenteral route (IV) will get the drugs into his system more quickly than the oral route. RE will probably also get a bronchodilator to treat his wheezing, delivered via the inhalation route.

The resident prescribes aerosolized isoetharine for RE. As you are administering the treatment, RE exhibits tingling in his fingers and tells you that his heart is racing. His heart rate increases to 130 beats/min. You stop the treatment and phone the resident. What is the likely cause of RE's reaction to the medication? What alternative would you suggest to the resident?

Answer: Remember the old lock-and-key theory of drugs and receptors? Well, isoetharine is sort of like a skeleton key—it matches with both beta-1 (stimulates the heart) and beta-2 (bronchodilation) receptor sites. You need to give a bronchodilator with a more complex chemical structure, so it will only match with the beta-2 receptors. This will give RE bronchodilation without cardiac side effects. A good choice would be albuterol (with an intermediate time-plasma curve).

RE is your patient again the next day. After his albuterol treatment, RE is feeling much better. His respiratory rate is 18 breaths/min; his heart rate is 84 beats/min; good color; less wheezing. RE comments that a lot of the medicine seems to be going out into the air and that he can taste it in the back of his throat. He asks you how much of the stuff really makes it into his lungs.

What do you tell him?

_____

_____

_____

_____

_____

Answer: 10%! He's right. He actually swallows most of the drug!

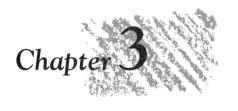

Chapter 3 Administration of Aerosolized Agents

Aerosol Therapy

Before we talk about how to give aerosol drugs, let's define *aerosol therapy*—it's the delivery of aerosol particles to the respiratory tract for therapeutic purposes. It's used for three things in respiratory care:

1. To humidify inspired gas (water aerosols)
2. To improve the mobilization and elimination of secretions—like a sputum induction (These aerosols can be water or saline.)
3. To deliver drugs to the respiratory tract (Remember the aerosol route of administration?)

Three other definitions are also important:

1. Stability—tendency of an aerosol to remain in suspension
2. Penetration—how far into the lung the aerosol particles go
3. Deposition—aerosol particles falling out of suspension

Q1. Which two of the above three definitions represent qualities that you would want in your "dream aerosol"? _____ _____ and

_____

Delivering drugs to the respiratory tract is the type of aerosol therapy we'll focus on in this chapter. The *advantages* to delivering drugs via the aerosol route follow:

1. Smaller doses can be used.
2. The drug acts quickly.
3. The drug goes right to the respiratory system.
4. There are fewer, less severe side effects (partly because of No. 1 above).
5. It's convenient and painless.

Disadvantages to this route include the following:

1. There are lots of factors that influence how much drug actually gets to the airways.
2. It's sometimes hard to estimate the right dose and/or you may not get the same dose every time.
3. It's hard for some people to coordinate depressing the canister and inhaling if they use an MDI. This is not such a big deal now that there are spacers (reservoir devices).
4. The health care practitioner may not know all that he or she should about the device that the patient is using and/or how to use that device. (But whose fault is that?)
5. There could be more technical info about aerosol therapy devices.

Q2. Quick! List two advantages and two disadvantages of aerosol drug delivery.

Advantages
1. _____
2. _____

Disadvantages
1. _____
2. _____

Here are some fun facts about aerosol particles!

1. Aerosol particles that are produced by MDIs, nebulizers, and DPIs come in many sizes—they're heterodisperse or polydisperse.

2. Aerosol particles are basically spherical.

3. You need to know what size the aerosol particles are, so that you can determine whether or not they'll make it into the airways or lung. Size is given using the mass median aerodynamic diameter (MMAD).

4. MMAD can be measured with a cascade impactor, which has a series of stages, each stage with a progressively smaller opening. A constant flow draws the particles through each stage. The biggest particles are collected on the first stage, etc. Any particles that make it through to the last stage get collected on a filter. Aerosol particles on each stage are measured by spectrophotometry.

5. The size of aerosol particles is one of the most important factors in determining whether the aerosol will get to the lung. Take a look at particle size and where the particles end up:

   - 10 to 15 µm gets stuck in the upper airway (nose and mouth). This might be good for nasal sprays.
   - 5 to 10 µm deposits in the upper airway.
   - 1 to 5 µm can make it to the lower respiratory tract. This is the appropriate size for the bronchoactive drugs that we use today.
   - 0.8 to 3 µm is likely to get to the lung parenchyma/alveoli. This is used for drugs where you don't want deposition in the larger airways because the effect is needed in the alveoli. (Pentamidine for treatment of human immunodeficiency virus [HIV] is a good example.)

𝒬3. Why is the size of the aerosol particle so important? _____
_____
_____

Three factors influence aerosol deposition in the lung:

1. Inertial Impaction—bigger particles, more turbulent flow, and higher velocities move faster, so they're more likely to run into something (like the pesky upper airway), and fall out of suspension.

2. Gravitational Settling—bigger particles that move slower are more likely to fall out of suspension due to the force of gravity.

3. Diffusion (Brownian Motion)—particles less than 1 µm in size may either be exhaled or just stay in suspension. (The time it takes for it to deposit anywhere is longer than a normal inspiration.)

How much aerosol actually gets to the lung periphery also depends on the patient's breathing pattern. Slow, deep breaths with an inspiratory hold, through the mouth are best.

𝒬4. Write down step-by-step instructions that you would give when instructing a patient on how to breathe during their med neb treatment. _____
_____
_____
_____
_____

Delivery Devices

Next, let's talk about the devices available to deliver aerosol therapy.

Nebulizers

All nebulizers have a reservoir chamber, baffle(s), and some way to shatter the liquid into gas suspension. Small volume nebulizers (SVNs) are the most common type used to deliver aerosol therapy. Here's what they look like:

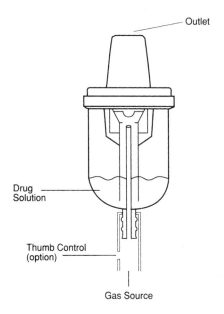

- They're pneumatic (gas powered).
- They have small reservoirs to hold the medication (hence, the name).
- Some have a thumb control, so that the patient only gets meds during inspiration.
- These devices are the most forgiving. You don't have to have great coordination or the perfect breathing pattern to use an SVN. You get your meds over 100 breaths instead of two or four, like the MDI.
- It's not perfect, though! You've got to keep it clean, it's bulkier and harder to lug around (more conspicuous) than the MDI, and you need a power source to run it.

You can also deliver aerosolized drug with intermittent positive pressure breathing (IPPB), but if the patient can breathe on his or her own, SVNs are a better choice. If you use an SVN with a mask instead of a mouthpiece, you should know that much less drug makes it to the lung—only about 1% to 2%. Eek!

*Q*5. So, what size particles should the SVN be producing to affect the small airways in the lower respiratory tract?

_____

Ultrasonic nebulizers (USNs) are electrically powered and work on the piezoelectrical principle. (Remember this for your board exams!).

- These nebulizers produce a dense, high output aerosol. They're nice to use for sputum inductions!
- The higher the frequency, the smaller the particle size produced.
- Portable USNs are nice because they're so small.
- The treatment doesn't take as long as with SVNs because the drug is nebulized faster.
- But (you knew this was coming) USNs are more expensive than SVNs, and you've got to have electrical power.

*Q*6. Compare the SVN with the USN. List an advantage of each. (An advantage of one automatically becomes a disadvantage of the other!)

SVN Advantage:

_____

_____

USN Aadvantage:

_____

_____

Small aerosol particle generator (SPAG) is a large reservoir nebulizer, used for long periods of nebulization. It's marketed for use with the drug ribavirin (used to treat respiratory syncytial virus). We'll go over the SPAG more when we discuss ribavirin (Chapter 13).

Since SVNs are the most common, there are some things you need to know about pneumatic nebulizers.

1. Dead volume—This is how much drug is left in the neb when it begins to make that sputtering noise, and no more mist comes out. This usually amounts to 0.5 to 1 ml. Some of the drug is also lost into the air during the treatment. Patients get from 35% to 60% of the drug before sputtering occurs.

Bottom line—be sure to rinse the neb after a treatment to get rid of the residue, If you don't, the patient will get a more potent treatment (with potentially more side effects) next time.

2. Reliability—All SVNs are not created equal! Be sure you're using a brand that doesn't leak, etc.

3. Filling volume and treatment time—The most efficient volume to nebulize is 3 to 4 ml. (More than this, and the treatment takes so long the patient may not do it; less than this and the neb doesn't perform as well—that dead volume gets reached pretty quickly.)

4. Flow rate—The best is 6 to 8 L/min. This keeps treatment time lower than 10 minutes, and gives you the best particle size.

5. Solution type—The guidelines that we just went over are appropriate for bronchodilators, but antibiotics and pentamidine have different viscosities and physical characteristics, so volumes and flows may need to be modified.

𝒬7. List the characteristics of the perfect nebulizer treatment.

Filling volume: _____
_____

Treatment time: _____
_____

Flow rate: _____
_____

Metered Dose Inhalers

Here's a picture and the general sequence of events that occur when you use an MDI:

METERED DOSE INHALER

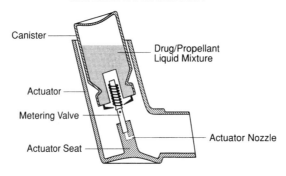

METERING VALVE FUNCTION

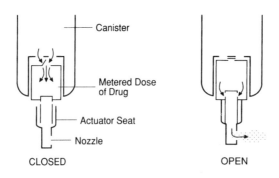

ADAPTERS

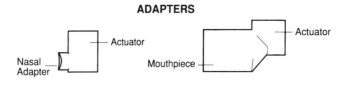

- The canister is depressed into the actuator.
- The mixture of propellant and drug is released under pressure.
- That mixture expands and vaporizes as it hits the air, which turns the liquid stream into an aerosol.
- When the canister is released, the metering valve refills with the drug-propellant mix and is ready for the next discharge.

The propellants are blends of liquefied gas chlorofluorocarbons (CFCs, freon).

The aerosol particle size depends on the vapor pressure of that propellant blend and the diameter of the actuator opening.

MDIs are soooo wonderful because they are portable and small, deliver aerosol drugs as efficiently as an SVN, and don't take long to administer.

On the flip side, you've got to be somewhat coordinated to use one, it's hard to tell when the canister is empty, a few patients may have a bad reaction to the propellant, and CFCs are released into the atmosphere. (This is a bad thing, environmentally speaking!)

And if you can believe this, one patient actually carried the MDI in his pocket without the cap on. A coin got stuck in the opening, and he actually aspirated it!

✐8. In your own words, write down how an MDI works.

_____
_____
_____
_____

To make sure that an MDI works optimally, pay attention to the following:

1. Don't store an albuterol canister in a valve-down position, Anywhere from 25% to 50% of the drug can be lost. If the MDI hasn't been used for 4 hours, discharge a waste dose.

2. Shake the MDI before you use it. Many of the drugs can separate from the propellant if it sits around.
3. Wait 30 seconds to 1 minute between puffs so that the dose output is not reduced.
4. If the MDI hasn't been used for days or weeks, propellant may be lost. Without propellant, little or no drug will be discharged. If the MDI hasn't been used for a long time, it should be shaken and a waste discharge should be given to prime the valve with drug and propellant.

Some people just can't coordinate depressing their MDI canister and breathing, so 3M Pharmaceuticals markets a breath-actuated inhaler. The canister is triggered by a spring that opens when the patient inhales.

As mentioned earlier, CFCs are not so hot for the environment. They cause damage to the ozone layer. Because of this, the United Nations Environment Program called for phasing out production of CFC by January 1, 1996. They also called for a ban on big hair, which required the use of hair spray propellant! Not.

CFC was hoarded so that it could be used until non-CFC propellants could be developed. A group of pharmaceutical companies have been working to develop these—they've discovered hydrofluorocarbons (HFCs). These propellants are not toxic to the atmosphere or the patient. That's a relief. Patients hate to breathe in toxic substances!

Some studies say that as many as 70% of people don't use their MDI correctly. Here's how to do it right:

- Assemble the inhaler and take off the cap.
- Shake the canister. (Remember to discharge a waste dose if it's been more than 24 hours since you used it last.)
- Open your mouth and hold the MDI about an inch away. If you can't do this, you can ask your doctor for a spacer device, or rest the mouthpiece on your lower teeth without closing your mouth around it.

- Exhale normally.
- Begin to take a slow deep breath through the mouth, pressing down on the canister as you continue to inhale. Breathe in until your lungs are full.
- Hold your breath for 10 seconds. (If you can't do 10, hold it as long as you can.)
- Exhale away from the mouthpiece.
- Wait 30 seconds before taking another puff.
- Don't forget to recap when you're done.

✐9. Your patient, Miss Scarlet, is being discharged from the hospital today. Please provide her with written instructions on how to properly use her MDI.

_____

_____

_____

_____

_____

It's a little different when you inhale a corticosteroid. Some patients get an infection in the back of their throats when they inhale a corticosteroid, so the second and third steps below are really important. (We'll cover this more later.)

1. If you are using a bronchodilator in addition to a corticosteroid, use the bronchodilator first and wait 1 to 2 minutes before inhaling the corticosteroid.
2. Always use a spacer (so you don't get deposition in the back of your throat).
3. Rinse your mouth with water after you're done.

The following apply for all inhalers:

- Rinse the mouthpiece every day to keep it clean.
- Soak the mouthpiece once a week in solution of one half white vinegar and one half water for 20 to 30 minutes. Don't forget to rinse it.
- You can check to see how full your canister is by floating it in water.

Metered Dose Inhaler Reservoir Devices

MDI reservoir devices are designed so that aiming the canister, coordinating hand and breathing, and depressing the canister would not be a problem.

Particles that come out of the MDI are about 35 μm. The reservoir allows enough time to vaporize to the point of 1 to 5 μm, so lung deposition is better.

There are many brands of reservoir devices. They're also called spacers, auxiliary devices, extension devices, holding chambers, add-on devices, etc. But what's in a name?

Technically, "spacers" don't have one-way valves to contain the aerosol until the patient is ready. If you know this fact, you will really impress your clinical instructor!

You can deliver 10% to 15% of the aerosol to the lung if you use good technique and a reservoir device.

✐10. One more time, what's the difference between a reservoir and a spacer?

_____

_____

Dry Powder Inhalers

A DPI is drug in powder form that comes in a small device and is breath actuated.

There are only two drugs available by DPI in the United States—cromolyn sodium (Intal) and albuterol (Ventolin Rotacaps). Before inhalation, a capsule is inserted into the Spinhaler or Rotahaler. The capsule is opened, and the patient inhales the very fine (by fine, I mean consistency) powder. These have been shown to be as effective as MDIs in drug delivery.

DPIs are good for the following reasons:

- They're small and easy to use.
- They contain no CFC propellants.

- It's easy to tell how much drug is left. (Count the capsules!)

Drawbacks to DPIs are as follow:

- There are only two drugs available this way.
- Some patients might react to the carrier substance.
- You've got to be able to generate an inspiratory flow of more than or equal to 60 L/min. (This may be hard for small children or asthmatic individuals in the midst of an attack.)

$\mathcal{Q}$11. List two advantages to DPI over MDI aerosol administration.

    1. _____
    2. _____

Since all the devices we've talked about deliver about the same amount of aerosol drug to the lung, how do you decide which one to use? Check out the box below:

We'll come back to this for the simulation after the NBRC-type questions.

1. Aerosol therapy is used for all but which of the following purposes?
    a. Humidification of inspired gases
    b. Improving mobilization and clearance of secretions
    c. Augmenting alveolar ventilation
    d. Delivery of medication

    (Chapter 3, p. 34)

2. Which of the following are advantages of delivering medication using the aerosol versus systemic route of administration?
    I.   Smaller doses are required.
    II. Onset of action is quicker.
    III. Side effects are fewer.
    IV. Drug delivery is targeted to the respiratory system.

    a. I, II, III, IV
    b. II, III
    c. III, IV
    d. I, II, IV

    (Chapter 3, p. 35)

Guidelines for the Differential Selection of Aerosol Delivery Devices

Nebulizer—use if an individual

- is unable to follow instructions or is disoriented
- has a poor inspiratory capacity
- is incapable of a breath-hold
- is tachypneic (>25 breaths/min) or has an unstable respiratory pattern
- needs to aerosolize a drug not in MDI or DPI form

Metered Dose Inhaler—use if an individual

- is able to follow instructions and demonstrate correct use
- has an adequate inspiratory capacity
- is capable of a breath-hold
- has a stable respiratory pattern
- needs a drug available in MDI form

Auxiliary (Spacer) Devices—use for individuals

- inhaling aerosolized corticosteroids
- with poor hand-breathing coordination in use of an MDI
- simply to enhance MDI use and reduce oropharyngeal loss, with all MDI aerosols

Dry Powder Inhaler—use for individuals

- if the drug is available in DPI form
- with poor MDI coordination
- sensitive to CFC propellants
- capable of high inspiratory flowrates (>60 L/min) for cromolyn or albuterol
- who need accurate dose count monitoring

3. Which particle size is optimal for aerosol deposition in the lower airways?
   a. >10 μm
   b. 5 to 10 μm
   c. 2 to 5 μm
   d. 0.8 to 3 μm   (Chapter 3, p. 37)

4. How should a patient be instructed to breathe during an aerosol treatment to achieve optimal drug deposition in the lower respiratory tract?
   a. Slow, deep
   b. Fast, shallow
   c. Slow, shallow
   d. Fast, deep   (Chapter 3, p. 39)

5. Which aerosol delivery device operates on the piezoelectrical principle?
   a. SVNs
   b. SPAGs
   c. DPIs
   d. USNs   (Chapter 3, p. 40)

6. Advantages of SVNs over other types of delivery devices include all but which of the following?
   a. Little patient coordination required
   b. Is not effective at low inspiratory flows
   c. Inspiratory pause not necessary for efficacy
   d. Is able to aerosolize any drug solution
                            (Chapter 3, p. 41)

7. Which of the following aerosol delivery devices requires the patient to be able to generate an inspiratory flow rate of 60 L/min or greater?
   a. USN
   b. SPAG
   c. MDI
   d. DPI   (Chapter 3, p. 52)

8. Which of the following is true regarding inhalation of a corticosteroid via MDI?
   a. Wait 3 minutes between inhalations.
   b. If a bronchodilator is prescribed, use it after the corticosteroid.
   c. Rinse the mouth and throat with water after inhalation.
   d. It is unnecessary to use a spacer device with a corticosteroid.
                            (Chapter 3, p. 48)

9. Which two drugs are currently available in DPI form?
   a. Albuterol and metaproterenol
   b. Salmeterol and albuterol
   c. Cromolyn sodium and isoetharine
   d. Albuterol and cromolyn sodium
                            (Chapter 3, p. 50)

10. How much of the total drug dose is delivered to the lung, regardless of the delivery device used?
    a. 10%
    b. 30%
    c. 50%
    d. >50%   (Chapter 3, p. 54)

Sim

Professor Plum, a 38-year-old white man with a history of asthma, presents to the emergency department with a chief complaint of shortness of breath. His respiratory rate is 34 breaths/min; he cannot hold his breath; he is wheezing on both inspiration and expiration and using accessory muscles. He complains of anxiety, and he is diaphoretic. The physician has prescribed albuterol and asks for your recommendation as to method of delivery. What do you recommend?

_____

_____

_____

_____

_____

Why did you make this selection?

_____

_____

_____

_____

_____

Answer: The most appropriate selection, based on the information given, is SVN. Professor Plum has a high respiratory rate, no breath-hold, and may be short of breath to the point where it is difficult for him to focus on instructions. SVN allows him to receive his medication over many breaths (>100), rather than 2 to 4 that would be prescribed with MDI. Remember, because the number of chances to deliver the medication is limited with MDI, good technique is crucial. DPI would be a bad choice for the same reasons, plus the professor may not be able to generate the necessary flow rate in the midst of his attack.

It is 24 hours later. The wheezing has subsided considerably, existing only slightly on expiration. Professor Plum has a respiratory rate of 20 breaths/min, states that he is not experiencing dyspnea, and is able to hold his breath for 5 seconds. Is he still a good candidate for albuterol via SVN? Why or why not?

_____

_____

_____

_____

_____

Answer: Go crazy and switch him over to MDI. (Remember, it's more cost effective and easy to use). His respiratory rate, inspiratory hold, and the fact that he's feeling better (no longer shortness of breath) make him a good candidate for MDI.

Does he need a reservoir device? Why or why not?

_____

_____

_____

_____

_____

Although it's not imperative that he use a reservoir device, it can't hurt. If your technique is off even a little bit, reservoir devices are great.

Chapter 4 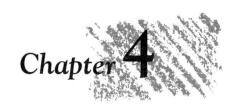 Calculating Drug Doses

In this chapter you will learn everything you ever wanted to know about drug dosage calculations. . . and more!

To do the calculations you've got to use the metric system—liters and grams.

And don't forget the Latin prefixes that go with them:

deci = 1/10
centi = 1/100 (cm, etc.)
milli = 1/1000 (mm, mg, etc.)
micro = 1/1,000,000

Not to leave out the Greeks:

deca = 10
hecto = 100
kilo = 1000

Practice a few conversions until you get the hang of it. If you already get it, skip it.

Q1. 51 cm = _____ mm
Q2. 33 g = _____ mg
Q3. 24 ml = _____ L
Q4. 17 m = _____ cm
Q5. 68 kg = _____ mg = _____ g

Here's an important piece of info. 1 g equals the weight of 1 m of distilled water at 4° C in vacuo. So 1 g is equal to 1 m, but it's only true when converting volume to volume. Don't use it to convert weight to volume. They're not always equal depending on the temperature and pressure of the substance.

In case you get an order for drops:

1 m = 16 gtts (drops)

Q6. How many drops in 3 m? _____
_____

Q7. How many drops in 0.5 m? _____
_____

1 cubic centimeter (cc) equals 1 m, so it's best to convert drops to milliliters and draw up your meds in a small syringe, like a tuberculin syringe. All drops are not created equal! The size of the opening and the properties of the liquid can influence the size of the drop.

Q8. A physician orders 2 drops of a medication. (It must be really potent!) How many milliliters is this?
_____

Calculating Doses From Prepared-Strength Liquids, Tablets, and Capsules

In this section you'll learn how to perform three types of calculations: (1) fluids, tablets, or capsules of a certain strength (mg/ml); (2) percentage strength solutions; (3) IV infusion rates. Make sure that you feel comfortable with metric conversions before you begin this section.

Calculating with Proportions

To do these calculations you're trying to figure out how much liquid, how many tablets, etc., you need to get the amount of drug that you want. There are two ways to do this. Use whichever one is easier for you.

1. Make sure you convert to consistent units of measure (grams to milliliters, drops to milliliters, etc.)!

2. Here's where you have a choice:
Set up a straightforward proportion:

$$\frac{\text{Original dose}}{\text{Per amount}} = \frac{\text{Desired dose}}{\text{Per amount}}$$

OR

Original dose: Per amount ::
Desired dose: Per amount

Let's take an example and work it both ways.

Divalproex is a drug used to treat migraine headaches. It is available in 500-mg tablets. A dosage of 1 g/day is prescribed for a patient. How many tablets should the patient take?

First, convert grams to milligrams: 1 g = 1000 mg.

You could probably do the rest in your head, but humor me so you get the sequence down.

The original dose is 500 mg (amount in 1 tablet).
Per amount = 1 tablet
Desired dose = 1000 mg
Per amount = x

So you can either do the following:

$$\frac{500 \text{ mg}}{1 \text{ tablet}} = \frac{1000 \text{ mg}}{x \text{ tablets}}$$

Remember algebra:

$$
\begin{aligned}
1000\,(1) &= 500\,(x) \\
1000 &= 500\,(x) \\
x &= 2 \text{ tablets}
\end{aligned}
$$

Let's say the percentage amount part changes (just to give you some challenge).

My kid's cough medicine contains 10 mg dextromethorphan hydrobromide in 5 ml. If the pediatrician tells me to give 3 ml, how many mg have I given?

Original dose = 10 mg; Per amount = 5 ml;
Desired dose = x; Per amount = 3 ml

Plug in the numbers:

$$\frac{10 \text{ mg}}{5 \text{ ml}} = \frac{x}{3 \text{ ml}}$$

$$
\begin{aligned}
10\,(3) &= (x)\,5 \\
30 &= (x)\,5 \\
x &= 6 \text{ mg}
\end{aligned}
$$

Drug Amounts in Units

There are certain drugs, like insulin and heparin, that come in units instead of milligrams or grams. You set up these types of problems exactly like the ones you just learned about.

Let's look at a common example.

Heparin often comes 1000 U/m. How many milliliters do you need to give to deliver 650 U of heparin?

1000 = original dose; 1 ml = Per amount;
650 Units = Desired dose; x = Per amount

$$\frac{1000}{1 \text{ ml}} = \frac{650}{x \text{ ml}}$$

$$
\begin{aligned}
1000\,(x) &= 650\,(1) \\
1000\,(x) &= 650 \\
x &= 0.65 \text{ ml}
\end{aligned}
$$

Insulin has a standard preparation:

$$0.04 \text{ mg} = 1 \text{ unit.}$$

Calculations with a Dosage Schedule

Sometimes, you have to calculate drug dosage from a schedule, based on a person's size.

For example, the average dose of sodium nitroprusside is 3 µg/kg/min. If you have a prepared strength vial of 50 µg/m, how much of that drug preparation should you give to a 70-kg man?

First, calculate the dose you'll need:

$$3 \text{ µg /kg} \times 70 \text{ kg} = 210 \text{ µg}$$

*Q*9. Quick! How many grams is that?

_____

Anyway, now calculate the amount of the preparation:

$$\frac{50 \ \mu g}{1 \ ml} = \frac{210 \ \mu g}{x \ ml}$$

$$50 \ (x) = 210$$

$$x = 4.2 \ ml/minute$$

It's too easy, isn't it!?

Let's do one more just for fun, though.

Let's say surfactant is administered at 5 ml/kg. You are asked to determine the dosage for a 1500-g premature infant.

First, convert grams to kilograms

$$1500/1000 = 1.5 \ kg$$

Next, multiply the recommended dose by kilograms:

$$5 \times 1.5 = 7.5 \ ml$$

There are more questions like this at the end of the chapter and also in the text.

Calculating Doses From Percentage Strength Solutions

Keep in mind these definitions:

Solution—*solute* dissolved in a *solvent*, resulting in a homogeneous mixture

Strength of solution—parts of active ingredient (solute) contained in 100 ml of the total solution (Solute + Solvent)

Types of Percentage Strength Preparations

Weight to Weight—grams of drug or active ingredient per 100 g of a mixture

Weight to Volume—grams of drug (active ingredient) per 100 ml of a mixture

Volume to Volume—ml of drug (active ingredient) per 100 ml of a mixture

Solution by Ratio

Often when you need to dilute medication to use in aerosol therapy, a solute-to-solvent ratio is given. For example, isoproterenol 1:200 or albuterol 1:12.

In the isoproterenol example 1:200 means 1 g/200 ml of solution.

$$1/200 = 0.005$$

which is 0.5% strength (0.005 × 100)

The albuterol example (ratio by simple parts) indicates actual parts medication to parts solvent. In this case 0.25 ml albuterol to 3 ml (0.25 × 12) normal saline gives you the 1:12 ratio.

The bad thing about this is that if the physician ordered just the ratio, and you didn't know that 0.25 ml was the usual dose of albuterol, you'd be out of luck.

Solving Percentage Strength Solution Problems

If you know that the active ingredient is 100% pure and not diluted, use this equation:

$$\begin{array}{c} \text{Percent strength} \\ \text{(in decimals)} \end{array} = \frac{\text{Solute}}{\begin{array}{c} \text{Total amount} \\ \text{(solute + solvent)} \end{array}}$$

If the active ingredient is diluted, use this equation:

$$\frac{\begin{array}{c} \text{Percent strength} \\ \text{(in decimals)} \end{array}}{\begin{array}{c} \text{Total amount} \\ \text{of solution} \end{array}} = \frac{\begin{array}{c} \text{Dilute solute x \%} \\ \text{Strength of solute} \end{array}}{\begin{array}{c} \text{Total amount} \\ \text{of solution} \end{array}}$$

Let's look at a couple of examples.

1. How many milligrams of active ingredient are there in 5 ml of 1:500 drug xyz? First, figure out the percentage strength (always do this first!)

$$1:500 = 0.002$$

Total amount of solution is 5 ml.

Active ingredient = x

Fill in the blanks from the equation above:

$$0.002 = x \text{ g}/5 \text{ ml}$$
$$x \text{ g} = 0.002 \times 5 = 0.01 \text{ g Active ingredient}$$

But wait. The question asked how many milligrams, so don't forget to convert!

$$0.01 \text{ g} = \underline{\hspace{2cm}} \text{ mg}$$

Answer: Yes, if you said 10, you're the big winner!

2. How much 10% Mucomyst do you need to prepare 6 ml of 20% Mucomyst? (This drug comes in these two strengths, and is used to liquefy secretions.) Because 10% and 20% indicate that Mucomyst is not 100% pure, you've got to use the equation for diluted active ingredient:

Percent strength (desired) = 0.20
Dilute solute (active ingredient) = x ml
% Strength of solute = 0.10
Total amount of solution = 6 ml

Plugging in these numbers to the appropriate equation:

$$0.20 = x \, (0.10) / 6 \text{ ml}$$
$$x \, (0.10) = 0.20 \times 6$$
$$x \, (0.10) = 1.2$$
$$x = 1.2/0.10 = 12 \text{ cc of 10\% Mucomyst}$$
(this treatment will last forever!)

Don't forget to give your answer in the units that are asked for in the question!

Don't forget to use decimals when solving % strength problems!

Don't forget to convert to metric units!

Which is more dilute—5 mg of active ingredient in 3 ml, or 5 mg active ingredient in 6 ml?

Answer: They're the same. You're delivering 5 mg of drug in both cases; the only difference is that the treatment will take longer to administer with more diluent added.

Calculating Intravenous Infusion Rates

This calculates the rate of drug administration per unit of time—like micrograms per minute.

There are basically two steps involved in doing these types of calculations:

1. Calculate how many milliliters per minute are needed.
2. Convert this flow rate (milliliters per minute) to drops per minute, using the standard drop factor. (You get this from the IV set.)

$$\text{Flow rate (ml/min)} = \frac{\text{Total solution (ml)}}{\text{Time (min)}}$$

$$\text{Flow rate (drops/min)} = \frac{\text{drops}}{\text{ml}} \times \frac{\text{ml}}{\text{min}}$$

If you need to deliver 1 L of IV solution for a period of 2 hours, what should be your flow rate in drops per minute, if the standard drop factor for your IV set is 15 drops/min? First, remember to convert (liters to milliliters, hours to minutes), and then just plug in the numbers.

$$x = \frac{15 \text{ drops}}{1 \text{ ml}} \times \frac{1000 \text{ ml}}{120 \text{ min}}$$

$$x = 15 \times 8.3 \text{ (because you can't give 8.3 drops, round this number: use 8).}$$

$$x = 15 \times 8 = 120 \text{ drops/minute}$$

Amount of Drug per Unit of Time

Some drugs need to be given in a certain concentration, like sodium nitroprusside (3 μg/minute). In these cases there's a giant equation you can use to plug everything in neatly:

$$\begin{array}{c}\text{Flow rate} \\ \text{(drops/min)}\end{array} = \frac{\text{Amount}}{\text{min}} \times \frac{\text{ml}}{\text{Amount}} \times \frac{\text{Drops}}{\text{ml}}$$

Try one:

What infusion rate do I need to deliver 5 µg/min of drug BC, which is available in a solution of 500 µg/1000 ml? Standard drop factor for your IV administration set is 15 drops/ml.

You know what to do next. Plug in!

$$\text{Drops/min} = \frac{5\ \mu g}{1\ \min} \times \frac{1000\ ml}{500\ \mu g} \times \frac{15\ \text{drops}}{1\ ml}$$

$$\text{Drops/min} = 5 \times 2 \times 15 =$$
$$150\ \text{drops/minute}$$

Following are 10 examples of calculations, written up á la NBRC. If you want more practice, there are 47 more in the text.

1. The RCP is asked to add 1 g of metaproterenol to 100 ml of aqueous solvent. This will result in which of the following concentrations?
   I.   1:1000
   II. 0.01%
   III. 1:100
   IV. 1%

   a. I and II
   b. II and III
   c. III and IV
   d. I and IV   (Chapter 4, p. 67-68)

2. You are asked to administer 1 ml of a 1% solution of isoetharine to an asthmatic patient. How many milligrams of drug is this?
   a. 1 mg
   b. 10 mg
   c. 100 mg
   d. 1000 mg   (Chapter 4, p. 67)

3. The physicians order reads, "Administer 5 mg metaproterenol via SVN." How many milliliters of a 1:100 solution should be used?
   a. 0.5
   b. 1
   c. 1.5
   d. 2   (Chapter 4, p. 68)

4. The RCP is asked to dilute 100 ml of a 2% solution of beclomethasone to a 1% solution. How many milliliters of water must be added to the original mixture to get the desired concentration?
   a. 100
   b. 50
   c. 200
   d. 150   (Chapter 4, p. 68)

5. How many milliliters of water are needed to dilute 10 ml of a 20% solution of acetylcysteine to a 5% concentration?
   a. 40
   b. 60
   c. 50
   d. 20   (Chapter 4, p. 68)

6. The physician's order reads, "Instill 5 ml 5% $NaHCO_3$ q4h and prn." All that the pharmacy has are 50 ml ampules of an 8.4% solution. How many milliliters of distilled water must be added to get a 5% solution?
   a. 10
   b. 21
   c. 34
   d. 42   (Chapter 4, p. 68)

7. The physician's order reads, "Administer 75 mg decadron via hand held nebulizer." How many milliliters of a 2.5% solution should you use?
   a. 2.2
   b. 0.5
   c. 3
   d. 1.5   (Chapter 4, p. 67)

8. You've got to get 1 L of normal saline into your patient at a drip rate of 15 drops/min. The standard drop factor of the IV set is 15 drops/ml. How long will it take to deliver it?
   a. 250 minutes
   b. 500 minutes
   c. 1000 minutes
   d. 1500 minutes   (Chapter 4, p. 71)

9. If you need to deliver 250 ml of solution during a 2-hour period, what drip rate should be set, assuming a standard drop factor of 15 drops/ml?
   a. 10 drops/min
   b. 30 drops/min
   c. 45 drops/min
   d. 50 drops/min   (Chapter 4, p. 71)

10. If a certain IV dose is ordered at 10 μg/min, how long will it take to reach the maximal dose of 0.65 mg?
    a. 32.5 minutes
    b. 65 minutes
    c. 97.5 minutes
    d. 130 minutes   (Chapter 4, p. 71)

Sim

A resident orders cromolyn sodium for one of your patients to be delivered via SVN. The drug is available as 20 mg in 2 ml of aqueous solution. What percentage strength are you delivering to your patient?

_____

_____

_____

_____

_____

You're doing a weight-to-volume calculation. Remember:

$$\text{Percent strength} = \frac{\text{Solute (in grams or ml)}}{\text{Total amount of solution}}$$

In this case first convert milligrams to grams:

$$(20 \text{ mg} = 0.02 \text{ g})$$

$$\% \text{ Strength} = 0.02 \text{ g}/$$
$$2 \text{ ml} = 0.01, \text{ or a } 1\% \text{ solution}$$

Chapter 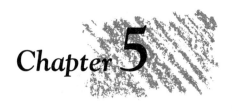 5 The Central and Peripheral Nervous System

In your body there are two major control systems—the nervous system and the endocrine system. I'm sure you've guessed from the title of this chapter that we're going to talk about the nervous system and how various drugs can manipulate it!

The nervous system is divided into (1) the *central nervous system* (CNS), which includes the *brain* and *spinal cord*, and (2) the *peripheral nervous system*, which includes the *sensory neurons*, *somatic neurons (motor control)*, and *autonomic nervous system (parasympathetic* and *sympathetic branches)*.

In case you've forgotten, the autonomic nervous system is the unconscious involuntary control mechanism that allows your body to function even when you're asleep or if you're in a coma. Let's look at its two branches:

Parasympathetic (PNS)	Sympathetic (SNS)
Essential to life	General alarm system—"fight or flight"
Finely regulated	Not essential to life
Controls digestion, bladder, rectal function	Increases heart rate, blood pressure, blood flow shifts from periphery to core

℘1. Give one example of when you'd want your SNS to be activated.

_____

_____

_____

_____

Neurotransmitters

To understand autonomic drugs, you've got to "get" neurotransmitters.

Neurotransmitters control nerve impulses.

Acetylcholine is the neurotransmitter everywhere (skeletal muscle, PNS terminal nerve sites, and all ganglionic synapses) except at SNS terminal nerve sites.

The autonomic nervous system is generally thought to be an efferent system. Quick! What's the difference between efferent and afferent nerve fibers?

Give up?

Efferent—impulses travel *from* the brain and spinal cord out to various sites (heart, lungs, Newark)

Afferent—impulses travel from the periphery *to* the spinal cord. Like when you touch a hot stove with the periphery (finger), and the "ouch" impulse gets sent to your brain—then out your mouth!

Following is a list of basic nervous system definitions that you really should know to impress your brain surgeon pals.

Parasympathomimetic—an agent *stimulating* the PNS (mimicking the action caused by acetylcholine at its receptor sites)—effect is bronchoconstriction

Parasympatholytic—an agent *blocking* the effects of the PNS (blocking acetylcholine)—effect is bronchodilation

Sympathomimetic—an agent *stimulating* the SNS (producing adrenergic effects)—effect is bronchodilation

Sympatholytic—an agent *blocking* the effects of the SNS (blocking adrenergic effects)—effect is bronchoconstriction

Cholinergic—a drug *stimulating* a receptor for acetylcholine

Anticholinergic—a drug *blocking* a receptor for acetylcholine

Adrenergic—a drug *stimulating* a receptor for norepinephrine or epinephrine

Antiadrenergic—a drug *blocking* a receptor for norepinephrine or epinephrine

2. Look these definitions over until you think you know them. Then try to match each term with its corresponding definition below. No cheating!
   a. agent blocking SNS
   b. agent stimulating PNS
   c. agent blocking epinephrine receptor
   d. agent blocking acetylcholine receptor
   e. agent stimulating SNS
   f. agent stimulating acetylcholine receptor
   g. agent blocking PNS
   h. agent stimulating epinephrine receptor

   _____ 1. sympathomimetic
   _____ 2. adrenergic
   _____ 3. parasympatholytic
   _____ 4. anticholinergic
   _____ 5. antiadrenergic
   _____ 6. parasympathomimetic
   _____ 7. cholinergic
   _____ 8. sympatholytic

Sympathetic Branch

When the sympathetic branch is activated, the following occur:

Stimulation of the heart	Increased cardiac output
Increased blood pressure	Mental stimulation
Accelerated metabolism	Bronchodilation

Remember, SNS stimulation is "fight or flight," so these signs are consistent with that phenomenon. Take a moment to think how each of the above would be an asset to you if you were in the "fight-or-flight" situation that you wrote down earlier. If you blew that off, pretend that your RT program director is chasing you around the lab with a long length of corrugated tubing because you hadn't completed this workbook properly!

Enzyme Inactivation

Chemicals that are structurally similar to epinephrine are called *catecholamines*. Two enzymes can inactivate them—sort of like how kryptonite inactivates Superman. Anyway, these enzymes are COMT (catechol O-methyl-transferase) and MAO (monoamine oxidase).

You see why they use the letters!

Certain bronchodilators that you'll give are catecholamines. This means that they're inactivated by COMT (mostly) and MAO. Because of this, their effects don't last very long.

Alpha and Beta Receptors

There are two types of sympathetic receptors (alpha and beta).

Stimulation of alpha receptors causes vasoconstriction. Stimulation of beta-1 receptors increases the rate and force of contraction of cardiac smooth muscle. Stimulation of beta-2 receptors causes bronchial and skeletal muscle relaxation.

Basically, alpha-1 and beta-1 receptors *excite*, and alpha-2 and beta-2 receptors *inhibit*.

On a continuum, phenylephrine is an almost pure alpha stimulant—epinephrine stimulates alpha and beta sites equally—isoproterenol is an almost pure beta stimulant.

Which site (alpha, beta-1, beta-2) would be best to stimulate if the patient had a runny nose?

_____

Answer: Alpha (vasoconstriction)—if you dilated the vasculature in the nose, the patient would be even more congested.

How about if you wanted to give relief to a patient in the midst of an asthma attack?

_____

Answer: Beta-2 (bronchial relaxation [dilation])

Neural Control of Lung Function

Both the PNS and SNS branches of the autonomic nervous system control lung function to some extent.

Airway Smooth Muscle

*Q*3. Although there's no *direct* sympathetic innervation of airway smooth muscle, the SNS controls smooth muscle tone by circulating epinephrine and norepinephrine. Norepi acts primarily on alpha receptors and epi acts on _____ receptors.

Lung Blood Vessels

The lung receives its blood supply from both the pulmonary (venous supply) and the bronchial (arterial supply) circulations.

Pulmonary circulation is innervated by both the PNS and SNS.

Arterial circulation is innervated mostly by the SNS.

Mucous Glands

Bronchial submucosal glands are innervated by the PNS and SNS. (When these glands are stimulated, you get lots more mucus! Hooray!)

Parasympathetic Innervation

The lung is supplied by vagus nerves that innervate the trachea. Branches of the vagus nerves innervate the hilum and smaller airways.

The vagus nerves release acetylcholine. (That's why they're called *cholinergic*.)

When acetylcholine combines with a certain receptor (muscarinic) on airway smooth muscle, you get bronchoconstriction. (When acetylcholine combines with a receptor on submucosal glands, you get more mucus.)

Acetylcholine is kept from going wild by an enzyme called cholinesterase, which breaks down acetylcholine.

A Tale of Acetylcholine

*Q*4. Once upon a time, acetylcholine was released by the _____ nerves. Acetylcholine combined with _____ receptors on _____ muscle, resulting in _____. When acetylcholine combined with receptors on _____, the result was more mucus. This all became a bit overwhelming, so in stepped the hero, _____, to calm down acetylcholine. The End

Select the best response to the following questions:

1. The SNS is part of which of the following?
   a. CNS
   b. Peripheral nervous system
   c. Autonomic nervous system
   d. b and c   (Chapter 5, p. 76)

2. Which branch of the nervous system controls daily functions like digestion and bladder control?
   a. CNS
   b. PNS
   c. SNS
   d. b and c   (Chapter 5, p. 76)

3. Which of the following describes a drug that stimulates the SNS?
   a. Parasympathomimetic
   b. Parasympatholytic
   c. Sympathomimetic
   d. Sympatholytic   (Chapter 5, p. 79)

4. Which of the following describes the autonomic nervous system?
   a. Sends impulses from the brain to the neuroeffector sites (heart, lungs)
   b. Sends impulses from the periphery to the brain and spinal cord
   c. Is exemplified by the knee-jerk reaction
   d. Is an afferent system
       (Chapter 5, p. 79)

5. Which of the following describes a drug that blocks a receptor for acetylcholine:
   a. Cholinergic
   b. Anticholinergic
   c. Adrenergic
   d. Antiadrenergic   (Chapter 5, p. 79)

6. SNS stimulation results in all but which of the following?
   a. Increased blood pressure
   b. Mental stimulation
   c. Increased urine output
   d. Bronchodilation   (Chapter 5, p. 86)

7. Which two enzymes inactivate catecholamines?
   a. TDH and BHG
   b. COTN and MNM
   c. DDT and TKO
   d. COMT and MAO
       (Chapter 5, p. 86)

8. Stimulation of which of the following receptors results in vasoconstriction?
   a. Alpha
   b. Beta-1
   c. Beta-2
   d. Gamma   (Chapter 5, p. 87)

9. Epinephrine accomplishes which of the following?
   a. Primarily stimulates alpha receptors
   b. Primarily stimulates beta receptors
   c. Stimulates alpha and beta receptors equally
   d. Stimulates neither alpha nor beta receptors   (Chapter 5, p. 90)

10. Blood flow to the lung is supplied by which of the following?
    I.   pulmonary circulation
    II. vagal circulation
    III. bronchial circulation
    IV. parasympathetic circulation

    a. I and IV
    b. II and III
    c. I and III
    d. II and IV   (Chapter 5, p. 92)

Sim

Methacholine is an inhaled parasympathomimetic agent used in bronchial challenge tests to determine the degree of airway reactivity in asthmatic individuals. What is the parasympathetic effect? How do you think methacholine might work to detect the degree of airway reactivity?

_____

_____

_____

Answer: The parasympathetic effect is bronchoconstriction. Parasympathomimetic drugs like methacholine are structurally similar to acetylcholine. They occupy cholinergic receptor sites at parasympathetic nerve terminals and cause activation of the receptor (bronchoconstriction). The more hyperreactive the airway, the greater the degree of bronchoconstriction in response to a certain dose of methacholine. A methacholine challenge is useful in determining the degree of airway reactivity between asthmatic and nonasthmatic individuals and also in assessing the severity of that reactivity.

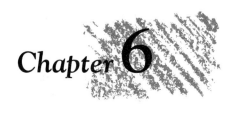

Chapter 6 Sympathomimetic (Adrenergic) Bronchodilators

This is probably the most important chapter in the whole book because inhaled adrenergic bronchodilators represent the most common drugs that you'll administer as a respiratory care practitioner.

They've been around for a long time, and the clear trend in development is toward agents that are more beta-2 specific (with little beta-1 effects). Now, circle either heart or lung in the next sentence. (Beta-2 specific means more of the desired effect on the (heart, lung) and less effect on the (heart, lung). Yes—we want more lung and less heart!

Following is a list of adrenergic agents given by inhalation (and some by other routes too). They appear in the order they were developed and also from least to greatest beta-2 specificity.

- Epinephrine (AsthmaNefrin, Primatene Mist, various)
- Isoproterenol (Isuprel)
- Isoetharine (Bronkosol)
- Metaproternol (Metaprel, Alupent)
- Terbutaline (Brethaire)
- Albuterol (Proventil, Ventolin)
- Bitolterol (Tornalate)
- Pirbuterol (Maxair)
- Salmeterol (Serevent)

$\mathcal{Q}$ 1. Which bronchodilator from the above list is the most beta-2 specific?

_____

The general indication for these bronchodilators is *relaxation of airway smooth muscle to reverse or lessen the degree of airflow obstruction.*

Diseases where this is necessary include asthma (all types), chronic bronchitis, and cystic fibrosis.

Mode of Action

Adrenergic drugs work by stimulating beta-2 receptors on bronchial smooth muscle. Some adrenergic drugs (at or near the top of the list above) also stimulate alpha and beta-1 receptors. Think back—back—to Chapter 5. What are the results of alpha and beta-1 stimulation?

Alpha (vasoconstriction; decongestion)
Beta-1 (increased heart rate and force of contraction)

These are not what we want! So beta-2 specific drugs are what we want for Christmas. We get the following:

- Relaxation of bronchial smooth muscle

Plus, as a bonus . . .

- Inhibition of inflammatory mediator release
- Stimulation of mucociliary clearance

It's like a 2-for-1 sale or something!
Let's discuss specific adrenergic agents.

Catecholamines

The following are words to live by, like the Boy or Girl Scout Pledge: All sympathomimetic bronchodilators are catecholamines or derivatives of catecholamines.

I know you must be dying to know the definition of a catecholamine. Well, it's a sympathomimetic amine, and it mimics the action of epinephrine. (Remember, equal alpha and beta stimulation?)

> Q2. What effects do you get with alpha stimulation?
>
> _____
> _____

> Q3. What effects do you get with beta-1 stimulation?
>
> _____

> Q4. You guessed it, beta-2 is up next.
>
> _____

Now we'll talk in a tad more detail about the drugs listed earlier, beginning with *epinephrine*. It's a potent catecholamine bronchodilator, but it also gives you alpha and beta-1 stimulation.

It works quickly (rapid onset) but doesn't last long because it's metabolized by COMT. (Remember that pesky enzyme?)

> Q5. It's better to use epinephrine for acute asthma episodes than for maintenance. Why?
>
> _____
> _____
> _____

You might hear of a drug called *racemic epinephrine*, which is a synthetic form of *epinephrine*. It also gives both alpha and beta effects, but with about half the vasoconstrictor effect. It's sometimes used to treat croup.

Isoproterenol is a pretty potent bronchodilator. (It has strong beta-1 and beta-2 effects.) When it first came out, everybody thought it was the greatest thing since the model-T, but now that there are drugs that are much more beta-2 specific, it's not used much as a bronchodilator. It doesn't last long either because of its breakdown by COMT.

> Q6. *Isoetharine* was one of the first beta-2 specific drugs available in this country. Because it's a catecholamine, the duration of action is _____ because it is inactivated by _____. It has a quick onset and few cardiac side effects, so it's sometimes used in pre-post bronchodilator studies.

I'll bet you're probably wishing that you knew just *how* those pharmacological geniuses actually made the catecholamines more beta-2 specific! Really, I know you don't care, so I'll be brief.

It's basically explained by the keyhole theory of beta sympathomimetic receptors. Cateholamines have a catechol base and an amine side chain (kind of like a key). The longer and more complex the side chain, the more beta-2 specific the drug. It's like a skeleton key will fit in many locks, but the intricate key to your BMW will only fit your car.

Don't forget that a limitation of all these drugs is that they are inactivated by COMT, found mainly in the liver and gut. All the drugs we've talked about so far only last $1\frac{1}{2}$ to 3 hours.

> Q7. This is probably obvious to you, but because catecholamines are inactivated in the _____ and _____, you really shouldn't give them orally!

Resorcinols were created by modifying the old catechol nucleus, so it would no longer be inactivated by COMT. What a triumph!

From this, we got *metaproterenol* and *terbutaline*. These are better than the unmodified catecholamines because they do the following:

- Last longer (up to 6 hours)
- Are beta-2 specific, with minimal cardiac side effects
- Can be taken orally (not vulnerable to COMT)
- Are slower to peak, which makes them a better choice for maintenance therapy

Saligenins resulted from a different modification of the catechol nucleus. An example is albuterol, which is available by mouth, MDI, aerosol, syrup, and DPI. They exhibit the same advantages over catecholamines as resorcinols, that are listed above.

Q 8. What are the advantages again?

_____

_____

_____

Pirbuterol (Maxair) is also a noncatecholamine adrenergic drug. You can only get it in MDI form. Onset of action is 5 to 8 minutes; peak effect occurs at about 30 minutes; it lasts about 5 hours.

Bitolterol: A Pro-Drug (Tornalate)

Bitolterol drug is called a pro-drug because you give it—it gets changed to something else in the body—and this becomes the active drug. But all the while, it's a catecholamine.

So, give the drug via MDI. It's gradually hydrolyzed by esterase enzymes. You get *colterol* (the active drug). Voila!

You get a sustained release effect, like the cold capsule on TV ads, so it lasts about 8 hours. Not bad. Remember, COMT will still inactivate colterol because it's a dyed-in-the-wool catecholamine. It just takes longer because of the gradual release.

Q 9. Bitolterol also has a bulky side chain, which means?

_____

_____

_____

Long-Acting Beta-Adrenergic Agents

The drugs that we've discussed so far share the limitation of lasting only 4 to 6 hours. This presents a problem for patients who need overnight control of their asthma. It's also easier for patients to take a pill or MDI two times a day than four times a day so this category of drugs might lead to better compliance.

There are two such drugs available—*sustained release albuterol* and *salmeterol.*

Sustained release albuterol is available as Proventil Repetabs or Volmax. Repetabs are pills that contain half the dose in the coating and half in the core, to be released after several hours. They last up to 12 hours.

Volmax is a pill that works on an osmotic gradient, pulling water into the tablet, dissolving the albuterol, and gradually releasing it through a pinhole in the tablet. Volmax can also last up to 12 hours.

Salmeterol is available via MDI, and it works differently than anything we've talked about yet. Its side chain is anchored at an exosite so that the active portion continually attaches and reattaches from the active beta receptor site. Cool. Anyway, this is how it lasts so long (12 hours, with a peak effect in 3 to 5 hours).

- Salmeterol also inhibits histamine for up to 20 hours—a definite plus! But don't use it as a substitute for corticosteroids.

The important thing to remember with the long-acting adrenergic drugs is do *not use them during an acute asthma attack!*

So you'll remember, write this 50 times. Okay, write it twice!

_____

_____

Q 10. Why is it a bad idea to use long-lasting adrenergic drugs during an acute asthma attack?

_____

_____

_____

_____

Salmeterol is used in patients who have asthma, need to use a beta agonist every day, and need to use inhaled corticosteroids or prophylactic agents to keep their asthma under control.

News flash! There are two drugs currently under investigation for the treatment of asthma whose effects may last 24 hours! They are formoterol and bamduterol.

*Q*11. The table below gives a list of the catecholamines and derivatives of catecholamines. (Repeat the mantra. All sympathomimetic bronchodilators are _____ or _____.) It also includes routes of administration, strength, and doses.

*Q*12. Remember, catecholamines are inactivated by _____, so they can't be given using the _____ route of administration.

Plus, inhalation is better because of the following:

- Fewer side effects
- Smaller doses
- More rapid onset—delivered directly to the lung
- Less pain and greater safety

*Q*13. What should you do if your patient is having trouble using an MDI correctly? Give the patient a _____.

What about giving beta agonists continually? Well, it's been done using a variety of methods (large volume nebulizers, refilling of SVN, volumetric infusion pumps) trying to treat severe asthma. These patients are very, very sick and need continuous monitoring.

Believe it or not, adrenergic bronchodilators have a few side effects. They vary between patients.

*Q*14. Remember, the more beta-2 specific the drug, the _____ side effects. Many of the side effects are dose related, so if your patient exhibits side effects at a certain dose, he or she may be fine if the dose is halved. Side effects include the following:

- Tremor
- Headache
- Increased blood pressure
- Dizziness
- Tolerance
- Hypokalemia
- Palpitations/tachycardia
- Insomnia
- Nervousness
- Nausea
- Worsened ventilation-perfusion ratio (decreased PaO_2)
- CFC-induced bronchospasm

Asthma mortality is on the rise in the United States, even though we have more treatment options than ever before. Here's why the experts think this may be happening:

- Beta agonists increase bronchial hyper-responsiveness.
- Patients develop tolerance to the bronchodilating effects of beta agonists.
- Patients overuse MDIs and don't get help as soon as they should.
- Patients with allergic asthma may allow themselves to be exposed to allergens without having any symptoms to warn them that they're getting in trouble.
- Patient education about and/or compliance with control of asthma with antiinflammatory drugs and beta agonists can be poor.

P.S. Don't use OTC medication to control asthma! Although, doesn't it look like you could drive a truck through the airways on the TV commercial?

The American Academy of Allergy and Immunology came out with a list of recommendations for the use of sympathomimetic bronchodilators. They're common sense, really. See if you can fill in the blanks based on what you've learned in this chapter.

𝒬 15. Beta agonists should be prescribed in _____ form whenever possible (minimal side effects, rapid onset).

𝒬 16. Patients should be monitored for adverse _____ side effects (result of beta-1 stimulation), especially if they are at risk for arrhythmias.

𝒬 17. OTC agents _____ be used to treat an asthma attack.

𝒬 18. If the patient has moderate asthma, the patient may also need _____ in addition to beta agonists to control asthma.

Here come the NBRC questions—I threw in a bonus question at no extra charge.

1. Which sympathomimetic bronchodilator is beta specific, but stimulates beta-1 and beta-2 receptors equally?
   a. Epinephrine
   b. Isoetharine
   c. Isoproterenol
   d. Salbuterol   (Chapter 6, p. 102)

2. Beta-2 receptor stimulation can have all but which of the following effects?
   a. Mucous gland hypertrophy
   b. Bronchial smooth muscle relaxation
   c. Inhibition of histamine release
   d. Stimulation of mucociliary clearance
                          (Chapter 6, p.103)

3. Catecholamines do which of the following?
   a. Mimic the action of catechol
   b. Mimic the action of epinephrine
   c. Have a prolamine nucleus
   d. Are alpha inhibitors
                          (Chapter 6, p. 105)

4. Which of the following describes catecholamines?
   a Long-acting
   b. Slow onset
   c. Useful for asthma maintenance therapy
   d. Inactivated by COMT
                          (Chapter 6, pp. 107-108)

5. Catecholamines are unsuitable for which route of administration?
   a. IV
   b. Inhalation
   c. Oral
   d. Subcutaneous   (Chapter 6, p. 108)

6. Metaproterenol is an example of which type of adrenergic bronchodilator?
   a. Catecholamine
   b. Resorcinol
   c. Saligenin
   d. Sustained release   (Chapter 6, p. 108)

7. Which of the following statements are true of bitolterol?
   I.   It is converted to colterol in the body.
   II. It is administered by tablet.
   III. Colterol is a catecholamine.
   IV. It can last up to 8 hours.

   a. I, II, III, IV
   b. I, II, III
   c. I, III, IV
   d. I, III, IV   (Chapter 6, pp. 109-110)

8. All but which of the following are side effects associated with the use of adrenergic bronchodilators?
   a. Worsening ventilation-perfusion
   b. Hypotension
   c. Nausea
   d. Tachycardia (Chapter 6, pp. 117-122)

9. Your patient is receiving metaproterenol 0.25 ml in 3 ml normal saline. Her heart rate increases from 80 to 120 beats/min. She complains of tremor and palpitations. What should you recommend to her physician?
   a. Initiate continuous nebulization
   b. Decrease the dose
   c. Switch to a drug with greater beta-2 specificity
   d. b or c   (Chapter 6, p. 132)

10. Which of the following catecholamines or catecholamine derivatives lasts the longest?
    a. Isoproterenol
    b. Terbutaline
    c. Metaproterenol
    d. Salmeterol   (Chapter 6, p. 105)

11. All but which of the following diseases is likely to respond well to adrenergic bronchodilators?
    a. Asthma
    b. Cystic fibrosis
    c. Chronic bronchitis
    d. Pulmonary fibrosis (Chapter 6, p. 102)

Sim

A 16-year-old patient suffers from moderate asthma. He is on a regimen of cromolyn sodium and corticosteroid. What would be the best choice of sympathomimetic bronchodilator to accompany this therapy?

_____

_____

_____

Answer: Salmeterol would be an excellent choice to accompany the prophylactic and anti-inflammatory agents because of its long-acting properties. A 16-year-old (or anybody else, I guess) is much more likely to comply with therapy the less often it has to be taken. He is already receiving both cromolyn sodium and a corticosteroid. Why prescribe a bronchodilator that has to be taken qid when a bid choice is available? Salmeterol is also a good choice because, since it lasts up to 12 hours, it can control asthma overnight.

Well, if it's so great, what is the one condition where it would be likely to cause your patient problems?

_____

_____

_____

Answer: If the guy (above) has an asthma attack, salmeterol is *not* the adrenergic bronchodilator of choice! Remember, it doesn't peak for 3 to 5 hours, so it won't give him any relief. And if he gets no relief, he may take another hit off the MDI—and another—until he experiences tachyphylaxis and cardiac side effects, which may result in death. This is nothing to play around with.

Chapter 7 Anticholinergic (Parasympatholytic) Bronchodilators

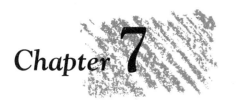

In this chapter we'll take a look at another class of bronchodilators—anticholinergics. They work by blocking ("anti") cholinergic-induced bronchoconstriction. This category of bronchodilators has also been around for a long time. People used to inhale fumes from the burning belladonna plant to treat respiratory disorders. Atropine is the original parasympatholytic.

Sympathomimetics pretty much replaced them as a primary treatment for asthma, but they're still around as an adjunct to therapy.

Ipratropium bromide (Atrovent) is the *one* anticholinergic aerosol to be approved for use as a bronchodilator in the United States (1987).

It's indicated for maintenance treatment of bronchoconstriction associated with chronic obstructive pulmonary disease (COPD).

Remember from Chapter 5 that PNS innervation maintains a certain level of muscle tone in the bronchi? This level of tone can be wiped out by anticholinergic agents, or intensified by cholinergic agents (methacholine) to the point of bronchoconstriction.

Anticholinergic agents block the action of acetylcholine. The effect will vary depending on the degree of tone (constriction) present that can be blocked.

Adrenergic bronchodilators act by causing relaxation of bronchial smooth muscle.

Q 1. Anticholinergic bronchodilators act by

_____

_____

_____ .

Vagally Mediated Reflex Bronchoconstriction

Some of the bronchoconstriction that occurs in patients with COPD is due to vagally mediated reflex innervation of bronchial smooth muscle. Here's what happens:

Sensory C-fibers → activated by stimuli → afferent nerve impulse response to CNS → reflex cholinergic efferent response causing bronchoconstriction, increased secretions, and cough.

Anticholinergic agents cause bronchodilation by preventing acetylcholine from causing bronchoconstriction.

Q 2. Circle one. Do parasympatholytics act (directly, indirectly) in causing bronchodilation?

Atropine is a *tertiary ammonium compound*. It gets absorbed by the blood stream, is distributed throughout the body, crosses the blood-brain barrier, and causes changes in the CNS.

Ipratropium bromide (Atrovent) is a *quaternary ammonium compound*. It is poorly absorbed, does not cross the blood-brain barrier, and does not cause CNS changes.

Q 3. Allright, Einsteins! Having read the above explanation of the difference between tertiary and quaternary ammonium compounds, which type do you think has greater systemic side effects?

_____

Since tertiary ammonium compounds have greater side effects, quaternary ammonium compounds, like Atrovent, are better choices for bronchodilation in the parasympatholytic class.

Onset of bronchodilation begins within minutes and peaks in 1 to 2 hours.

In asthma, ipratropium lasts about as long as a beta agonist (remember Chapter 6?) but in COPD, ipratropium lasts 1 to 2 hours longer.

The following are anticholinergic effects:

- Increased heart rate
- Drying of upper airway
- Urinary retention
- Mucociliary slowing
- Inhibition of constriction (this is your favorite)
- Dilated pupils (but not instructors!)
- Inhibited tear formation
- Constipation

Q 4. Compared to tertiary ammonium compounds, quaternary ammonium compounds, like _____, have the anticholinergic effects listed above to a (greater, lesser, same) extent. Cardiac and CNS system side effects usually don't occur with quaternary ammonium compounds.

CNS effects occur only with tertiary ammonium compounds. The CNS effects include the following:

- Restlessness
- Drowsiness
- Mild excitement
- Irritability
- Fatigue

With higher doses CNS effects include disorientation, hallucination, or coma. (Yikes! Those are bad.)

Let's take a look at the two parasympatholytic bronchodilators you'll be most likely to use.

Atropine Sulfate

Q 5. Atropine sulfate is a _____ compound, delivered via nebulized solution.

Both the incidence of side effects and duration are dose dependent.

Q 6. If I increase the dose, I _____ the likelihood of side effects and _____ the duration of bronchodilation.

In a dose necessary to achieve bronchodilation, side effects do occur.

Usual adult dose is 0.025 mg/kg tid or qid; onset occurs in 15 minutes; peak effect is seen in 0.5 to 1 hour; duration of effect is 3 to 4 hours.

Ipratropium Bromide

Q 7. Ipratropium bromide is a _____ compound. It's available as MDI (18 µg/ puff at 2 puffs qid), or nebulized solution (0.02% strength, which amounts to 500 µg tid or qid).

Onset for SVN is 1 to 5 minutes; duration is 4 to 8 hours.

Onset for MDI is 15 minutes; duration is 4 to 6 hours.

Q 8. Compare doses between MDI and SVN. How many micrograms are being given during one MDI treatment? _____ How many micrograms are being given during one SVN treatment? _____

Q 9. Which delivery route do you think is associated with greater incidence of side effects? _____

Common side effects for either method include cough and dry mouth.

For MDI, side effects (palpitation, rash, dizziness, nervousness, irritation, headache) occur occasionally.

For SVN, flulike symptoms, pharyngitis, dyspnea (that's not good!), bronchitis, nausea, occasional bronchoconstriction, and eye pain may occur. You've got to be careful in patients with glaucoma.

There's an MDI on the market called Combivent that combines albuterol and ipratropium, with the usual doses of each. It seems to be more effective in patients with COPD than either albuterol or ipratropium therapy alone. Neato.

Clinical Application

Take a look at the table below. It compares the general clinical effects of anticholinergic and beta-adrenergic bronchodilators.

	Anticholinergic	Beta-Adrenergic
Onset	Slightly slower	Faster
Time to peak effect	Slower	Faster
Duration	Longer	Shorter
Tremor	None	Yes
Fall in PaO_2	None	Yes
Tolerance	None	Yes
Site of action	Larger, central airways	Central and peripheral airways

Chronic Obstructive Pulmonary Disease

Anticholinergic bronchodilators seem to have their greatest effect on the central airways. They are more potent bronchodilators than beta-adrenergic bronchodilators in the bronchitis-emphysema combo. This is their primary clinical application.

Studies have shown improvement in baseline lung function with the use of ipratropium.

Use in Asthma

Anticholinergic bronchodilators aren't really better than beta-adrenergic bronchodilators in the treatment of asthma. But they might be useful if the patient has side effects with another class of bronchodilator or if patients need to be treated with beta blockers (patients with hypertension).

Combination Therapy: Beta-Adrenergic Plus Anticholinergic Agents

The combination of beta-adrenergic agents and anticholinergic agents could provide a one-two punch for patients with COPD or asthma because of the following:

1. Anticholinergics act primarily on the central airways; beta agonists act primarily on the peripheral airways.

2. Mechanisms of action are complementary.

3. Beta agonists peak quicker, but don't last as long (especially in patients with COPD); anticholinergics peak more slowly and last longer.

Q10. Beta-adrenergic agents cause
_____; anticholinergics block _____.

Q11. The combination drug, Combivent, is
_____ and _____.
Combivent is (more, less, equally) effective than either drug used alone.

Hasn't time flown since we began this chapter? I know you're shocked to learn that NBRC questions are next.

1. Which of the following is the only anti-cholinergic drug currently approved for use in the United States as an aerosolized bronchodilator?
   a. Atropine
   b. Belladona
   c. Ipratropium bromide
   d. Tertiary ammonium compounds
   (Chapter 7, p. 128)

2. Anticholinergic agents competitively block the action of which of the following substances?
   a. Catechol
   b. Sympathomimetics
   c. Beta-adrenergic agents
   d. Acetylcholine (Chapter 7, pp. 128-129)

3. All but which of the following are true of tertiary ammonium compounds?
   a. An example is ipratropium bromide.
   b. An example is atropine.
   c. They are associated with more CNS side effects than quaternary ammonium compounds.
   d. They are associated with more cardiac side effects than quaternary ammonium compounds.
   (Chapter 7, p. 133)

4. Which of the following describes quaternary ammonium compounds?
   a. Cross the blood-brain barrier
   b. Are easily absorbed
   c. Do not cause CNS changes
   d. Are distributed throughout the body
   (Chapter 7, p. 134)

5. Atropine sulfate is available in which of the following forms?
   a. Tablet
   b. Nebulized solution
   c. MDI
   d. b and c   (Chapter 7, p. 135)

6. Ipratropium bromide is available in which of the following forms?
   a. Capsule
   b. Nebulized solution
   c. MDI
   d. b and c   (Chapter 7, p. 135)

7. Which of the following are the most common side effects associated with administration of anticholinergic agents?
   I.   Cough
   II. Wheezing
   III. Dry mouth
   IV. Vomiting

   a. I, II, III, IV
   b. I and III
   c. II and IV
   d. I, II, III   (Chapter 7, p. 136)

8. Combivent is a combination of which two drugs?
   a. Metaproterenol and atropine
   b. Albuterol and atropine
   c. Metaproterenol and ipratropium
   d. Albuterol and ipratropium
   (Chapter 7, pp. 138-139)

9. Which is most effective in the treatment of COPD?
   a. Anticholinergic agents
   b. Beta-adrenergic agents
   c. a and b
   d. Alternate-day therapy
   (Chapter 7, p. 137)

10. In comparing anticholinergic and beta-adrenergic agents, anticholinergic agents are associated with which of the following:
    a. Faster onset
    b. Quicker time to peak effect
    c. No development of tolerance
    d. Shorter duration of action
    (Chapter 7, p. 137)

Sim

Jane COPD has a 122 pack per year smoking history. She suffers from a combination of emphysema and chronic bronchitis. Go figure! Lately, she's been more short of breath than usual, and her dyspnea is accompanied by some expiratory wheezing. What do you think she'll respond better to—sympathomimetic bronchodilators or anticholinergic bronchodilators? Justify your selection.

Answer: Hopefully, you didn't pick one. Trick question! The answer is the combination albuterol and ipratropium. Aha! You should select it for the following reasons:

Anticholinergic	Beta-Adrenergic
Acts on central airways	Acts on smaller airways
Peaks more slowly	Peaks sooner
Lasts longer	Terminates sooner

All these effects are complementary, for the longest lasting relief.

However, if you were forced to pick one of the above for Jane, choose anticholinergic agents. These have been proven to have at least somewhat of an impact on improving airflow. Some patients with COPD may suffer bothersome side effects as a result of adrenergic bronchodilators anyway, since many of these patients have heart difficulties.

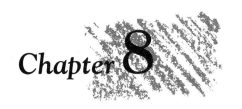

Chapter 8 Xanthines

Nobody is really absolutely sure how xanthines work, which makes it nice for you. (There's less to learn!) Xanthines are generally thought of as second- or third-string drugs in treating asthma and COPD.

Theophylline and caffeine are both methylxanthines. (The *methyl* part comes from having a methyl attachment to their chemical structure.)

General Pharmacological Properties

Following are the physiological effects of xanthines. These are easy to remember if you associate them with how you feel after drinking a large coffee, Surge, or Mountain Dew:

- CNS stimulation
- Cardiac muscle stimulation
- Cerebral vasoconstriction
- Diuresis
- Bronchial and vascular smooth muscle relaxation
- Peripheral and coronary vasodilation

Can you not identify with the increased heart rate, stimulatory effect, and diuretic effect?

If you compare theophylline and caffeine, although they exert the same effects, they do so to varying extents. Caffeine has greater CNS and skeletal muscle stimulation; theophylline provides a greater degree of cardiac stimulation, diuresis, and smooth muscle relaxation.

Q 1. Keeping the above comparison in mind, list one instance when caffeine and its physiological benefits would be of use to you; then do the same for theophylline.

Caffeine:

_____

Theophylline:

_____

Clinical Uses

Historically, theophylline has been used to treat asthma, COPD, and apnea associated with prematurity. Premature infants, that is—not your old boyfriend. That's *immaturity*.

Aminophylline has been used in treatment of asthma, but it's irritating to the pharynx, has a bitter taste, and can cause coughing and wheezing. Whose bright idea was it to treat asthma with a drug that causes coughing and wheezing?

Even though it's classified as a bronchodilator, it's a weak one compared to the beta agonists.

Q 2. In the treatment of asthma, rank the following classes of bronchodilators from most to least effective (1 is most effective):

_____ anticholinergic agents
_____ beta agonists
_____ xanthines

Q 3. How about treatment of COPD?

_____ xanthines
_____ anticholinergic agents
_____ beta agonists

Mode of Action

Nobody really knows how xanthines work. Xanthines may actually strengthen the diaphragm; they may inhibit phosphodiesterase (an enzyme), causing an increase in cyclic adenosine monophosphate (cyclic AMP), causing bronchodilation. Anyway, don't worry about it.

Titrating Theophylline Doses

People metabolize theophylline at different rates, so it's tough to determine a therapeutic dose. Plus, different forms of the drug aren't always equal, so this makes it even more difficult.

The optimal serum theophylline level for maximal bronchodilation in adults is believed to be between 10 and 20 µg/ml. More or less than that, here's what happens (usually):

Micrograms/milliliters	Effect
<5	none
10 to 20	therapeutic range
>20	nausea
>30	cardiac dysrhythmias
40 to 45	seizures

Since the 10- to 20-µg/ml range was proposed 25 years ago, it has been narrowed somewhat. (5 to 15 µg/ml is now recommended for the treatment of asthma; 10 to 12 µg/ml, for treating COPD.)

𝒬4. What is the therapeutic serum theophylline range for asthma?

_____

𝒬5. For COPD?

_____

𝒬6. What happens if the serum level is too low?

_____

𝒬7. So what do you do in that case?

_____

Dosage Schedules

Because of the variable rate at which people metabolize theophylline, dosage schedules are used to titrate it.

For rapid administration in an acute situation, 5 mg/kg _lean body weight_ should be given.

For long-term therapy, give an initial dose of 16 mg/kg/24 hr or 400 mg/24 hr, whichever is less.

𝒬8. Your patient weighs 60 kg. What theophylline dose should be given for long-term administration? _____

Even though you have properly calculated the dose, your patient complains of nausea.

𝒬9. What do you do? _____

Doses of theophylline should be guided by clinical reactions _and_ serum drug levels.

When drawing a blood level, get it 1 to 2 hours after administration of theophylline for immediate release forms and 5 to 9 hours after the morning dose for sustained release forms.

Theophylline Toxicity and Side Effects

A large problem with the use of theophylline is its narrow therapeutic range. Very little difference exists between the dose that will be therapeutic and the dose that will cause toxic side effects.

Q 10. Even if you stay in the therapeutic range (_____), you may experience side effects. The most common ones appear below:

CNS	Gastrointestinal	Respiratory	Cardiovascular	Renal
Headache	Nausea	Tachypnea	Palpitations	Diuresis
Anxiety	Vomiting		Supraventricular	
Restlessness	Anorexia		tachycadia	
Insomnia	Abdominal pain		Ventricular	
Temor	Diarrhea		arrhythmias	
Convulsions	Hematemesis		Hypotension	
	Gastroesophageal			
	reflux			

CNS, Central nervous system.
Effects are not listed in order of severity or progression.

If patients have excessive amounts of sputum (as occurs in cystic fibrosis, bronchiectasis, chronic bronchitis), be careful of theophylline's diuretic effect.

Q 11. What precautions might you take for these patients to make sure their sputum was fluid?

_____
_____
_____
_____

Factors Affecting Theophylline Activity

Theophylline is metabolized in the liver and eliminated by the kidneys, so any condition that affects these organs can affect theophylline levels. Serum levels are also affected by certain interactions with other medications.

Drugs that will *increase* blood levels of theophylline include beta blockers, corticosteroids, influenza virus vaccine, and estrogen.

Conditions that will *increase* blood levels of theophylline include hepatitis, renal failure, pneumonia, and congestive heart failure (CHF).

Drugs that will *decrease* serum theophylline levels include barbiturates, beta agonists, rifampin, and nicotine.

Clinical Application

As mentioned earlier, theophylline is not the drug of choice for maintenance of asthma or COPD. In can, however, be used for maintenance therapy in COPD if ipratropium bromide and beta agonists can't control the disease. As far as asthma, the American Thoracic Society suggests that theophylline only be used to provide relief *after* beta agonists, corticosteroids, and prophylactic agents have been implemented to target the underlying inflammation.

Q 12. If your patient consumes a lot of caffeinated beverages/foods while taking theophylline, he or she may experience side effects. What are these again? (I'm so forgetful!)

_____
_____
_____
_____

Nonbronchodilating Effects of Theophylline

Who cares if theophylline has bronchodilator effects! Just look at all the great nonbronchodilating action features it's got! The nonbronchodilating effects of theophylline include the following:

1. Respiratory Muscle Strength—Theophylline has actually been shown to increase the strength of the diaphragm! Who knew?

2. Respiratory Muscle Endurance—Theophylline prevents diaphragmatic fatigue.

3. Central Ventilatory Drive—Theophylline increases ventilatory drive at the CNS level, in particular, increasing phrenic nerve activity.

4. Cardiovascular Effects—Theophylline increases cardiac output, decreases pulmonary vascular resistance (PVR), and improves myocardial muscle perfusion. Wow!

5. Antiinflammatory Effects—In patients with allergic asthma, theophylline weakens the late phase to histamine.

As if this news isn't wonderful enough, the NBRC questions are next!

1. Theophylline is chemically referred to as one of which of the following?
   a. Beta blockers
   b. Anticholinergics
   c. Methylxanthines
   d. Aminophylline agonists
   (Chapter 8, p, 142)

2. Xanthines exhibit all but which of the following physiological effects?
   a. Bronchial smooth muscle relaxation
   b. Cerebral vasodilation
   c. Coronary vasodilation
   d. Diuresis   (Chapter 8, p. 142)

3. Compared with the beta agonists, theophylline has what degree of bronchodilating effect?
   a. Weak
   b. Comparable
   c. Strong
   d. Very strong   (Chapter 8, p. 143)

4. Which of the following make it difficult to titrate theophylline doses?
   I.   Theophylline has a short half-life.
   II. Theophylline is metabolized differently in individuals.
   III. Different forms of theophylline are not always equal.
   IV. The therapeutic range varies widely between patients.

   a. I, II, III
   b. II and III
   c. II and IV
   d. I, III, IV   (Chapter 8, pp. 145-147)

5. In the management of asthma, the therapeutic range for serum theophylline is which of the following?
   a. 2 to 12 µg/ml
   b. 5 to 15 µg/ml
   c. 20 to 30 µg/ml
   d. >30 µg/ml   (Chapter 8, p. 146)

6. Cardiovascular side effects associated with theophylline use include all but which of the following?
   a. Hypotension
   b. Ventricular dysrhythmias
   c. Supraventricular tachycardia
   d. Atrial dysrhythmias
   (Chapter 8, p. 147)

7. Which of the following can affect serum theophylline levels?
   I. Nicotine
   II. Influenza virus vaccine
   III. Hepatitis
   IV. Corticosteroids

   a. I, II, III, IV
   b. I, II, III
   c. II, III, IV
   d. I, III, IV   (Chapter 8, p. 148)

8. Nonbronchodilating effects of theophylline include all but which of the following?
   a. Increased diaphragmatic strength
   b. Increased phrenic nerve activity
   c. Decreased systemic vascular resistance
   d. Increased cardiac output
                                    (Chapter 8, p. 149)

9. Aminophylline was unsuccessful in the treatment of asthma because of which of the following?
   a. It caused the release of SRSA.
   b. It led to hypotension.
   c. It caused coughing and wheezing.
   d. It resulted in tolerance and tachyphylaxis.   (Chapter 8, p. 149)

10. Theophylline may be used to treat all but which of the following?
   a. Pneumonia
   b. Apnea of prematurity
   c. COPD
   d. Asthma   (Chapter 8, p. 149)

Sim

Joe COPD (no relation to Jane from Chapter 7) has been recently diagnosed with COPD. He is 57, has worked in the coal mines since he was 17, and suffers from severe dyspnea. Joe's physician prescribed oxygen for home use at 2 L/min, beta agonists, and corticosteroids. Joe has not responded as his physician had hoped. (There has been no change in his forced expiratory volume in 1 second [FEV-1]). She has decided to initiate sustained release theophylline for Joe, and asks you to calculate the appropriate dose for him. He weighs 75 kg and is 6 feet tall. What dose should you begin with?

_____

Answer: For long-term therapy, use 16 mg/kg/24 hr or 400 mg/24 hr, whichever is less. Joe's calculated dose is $16 \times 75 = 1200$ mg. Therefore 400 mg is less. (Yes, I am a rocket scientist!) So give him 400 mg the first day, which is 200 mg bid.

The following day, Joe feels no improvement, suffers no ill effects. You need to check a theophylline level. When is the best time to do this?

_____

Answer: 5 to 9 hours after the morning dose.

His level comes back 5 μg/ml. What do you recommend?

_____

Answer: Since Joe's clinical presentation is unchanged and his level is low (you want 10 to 12 μg/ml), recommend to his physician that his dose be increased, and monitor him closely.

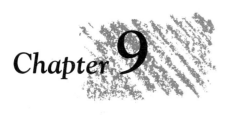

Chapter 9 Mucus-Controlling Drug Therapy

Aren't you excited to begin the study of mucus?! We'll take a fascinating look at the nature of mucus and how you can move it out using various drugs.

You probably already know that the mucociliary escalator (third floor—mucus glands) is one of the lung's primary defense mechanisms. If this system breaks down, you get thick secretions (airway obstruction).

Diseases that are associated with abnormal function of the mucociliary escalator include cystic fibrosis, chronic bronchitis, bronchiectasis, and asthma.

Mucus is a gel, with physical properties of viscosity and elasticity. Drug therapy is aimed at optimizing the *physical* state of mucus to move it up and out. Drugs in this category are called *mucus-controlling* or *mucoactive*.

Physiology of the Mucociliary System

The mucociliary system lines all the conducting airways, the nasal cavity, and the oropharynx. The system's got two layers: the sol layer on the bottom and the gel layer on top.

Types of cells that are responsible for secreting mucus include surface epithelial and subepithelial cells.

Surface Epithelial Cells

The surface of the trachea and bronchi includes ciliated cells and goblet cells in about a 5:1 ratio.

*Q*1. This means that for every single goblet cell, there are _____ ciliated cells.

There are 6800 goblet cells per square millimeter in the normal airway. Won't this be good info to share at the next party you go to?

*Q*2. So how many ciliated cells per square millimeter? _____

Subepithelial Cells

Submucosal glands make goblet cells look like big sissies in the mucus-producing area! They produce about 40 times more. These glands respond to cholinergic stimulation by increasing production of mucus.

Following are a few definitions, all of which your mucous vocabulary should not be without!

Mucus—total secretions from mucous membranes

Sputum—mucus plus saliva

Mucoactive—any agent (007) that affects mucus secretion

Mucolytic—breaking down the structure of mucus

Mukokinetic—improving mobilization and clearance of mucus

Expectorant—agent improving the ability to spew—no—agent improving expectoration of respiratory secretions usually by stimulating bronchial gland output

*Q*3. You knew it was coming—matching! Go crazy, you know what to do.
   a. all secretions from mucous membranes
   b. improving secretion mobilization
   c. stimulating the output of bronchial glands
   d. mucus plus saliva
   e. breaking down mucus
   f. affecting mucus

_____ 1. mucolytic
_____ 2. sputum
_____ 3. mucoactive
_____ 4. mucokinetic
_____ 5. expectorant
_____ 6. mucus

Ciliary System

Beating cilia move the mucous gel along. There are about 200 cilia on each teensy (5-μm) cell in the airway. The beat of a cilium is made up of a power stroke and a recovery stroke. They're like little synchronized swimmers!

Factors Affecting Mucociliary Transport or The Tortoise and the Mucus

Are you dying to know how fast mucus moves? 1.5 mm/min in peripheral airways, and 21.5 mm/min in the trachea. The following conditions make it move slower:

- Age greater than 56
- COPD
- General anesthetic
- Parasympatholytics
- Atmospheric pollutants
- Narcotics
- Endotracheal suctioning/tracheostomy

- Cigarette smoke
- Hyperoxia and hypoxia

*Q*4. Construct the *worst* possible patient and conditions for speedy mucus moving, using the list above.

_____
_____
_____
_____

As an aside, have you ever heard, "Milk makes mucus"? There are *no* scientific data to support this! I thought you needed to know.

Nature of Mucus Secretion

Healthy people produce about 100 ml of mucus every day, which just gets reabsorbed in the bronchial mucosa. About 10 ml of that reaches your glottis. You swallow or aspirate it without even flinching! Gag me. If you have bronchitis or pneumonia, you produce more secretions than usual, and they either get swallowed or expectorated.

Beta-adrenergic and methylxanthine agents increase ciliary beat, mucus production, and the transport of mucus.

*Q*5. Anticholinergic drugs decrease all that stuff (_____ _____).

*Q*6. Cromolyn sodium and corticosteroids have no effect on ciliary beat, _____ _____, or mucus transport.

Structure and Composition of Mucus

Mucus has a polypeptide (protein) backbone, formed by a string of amino acids. Carbohydrate side chains are attached to the amino acids.

Mucus forms a flexible strand that is cross-linked with disulfide bond. If disulfide and hydrogen bond, it can get even more cross-linked. You get a spongey gel with a high water content. It's like Jell-O. You've got to have enough water to make it in the first place. But once it's made, water doesn't get absorbed into the Jell-O. It rolls off of it.

Q7. Draw a diagram of mucus!

Mucus in Disease States

Certain diseases produce too much mucus. It's difficult to get rid of it all. Patients are more likely to come down with a bacterial infection. The mucus gets thicker. Ciliary motion becomes slowed or stops altogether. Airflow resistance can increase because of airway obstruction. Atelectasis may result.

Diseases that produce too much mucus include the following:

- cystic fibrosis
- asthma
- chronic bronchitis
- acute bronchitis

Q8. Describe the sequence of events that occurs when there's too much mucus!

_____

_____

_____

_____

Therapy for diseases that are characterized by hypersecretion of mucus should include the following:

1. Prevention—Stop smoking and avoid pollutants.
2. Optimize bronchial clearance—Drink plenty of fluids, cough and deep breathe, perform postural drainage, take bronchodilators and mucolytics as prescribed.
3. Treat inflammation—take corticosteroids as prescribed; treat infections early.

What's the difference between viscosity and elasticity?

Viscosity—resistance of a fluid to flow

Elasticity—ability of a deformed material to return to its original shape (like Stretch Armstrong or Silly Putty)

Q9. Which has higher viscosity—water or tomato sauce? _____

Q10. Which has greater elasticity—a rubber band or dough? _____

Answer: Well, tomato sauce has a higher resistance to flow (it doesn't flow as fast), so it has higher viscosity. And dough doesn't spring back to its original shape like a rubber band does! That's why schoolchildren don't flick balls of dough at each other.

Mucus-Controlling Agents

Acetylcysteine and dornase alfa are both mucolytic. Acetylcysteine breaks the disulfide bonds in mucus; dornase alfa breaks down DNA in airway secretions.

Acetylcysteine (Mucomyst)

Indications

Duh, it's used if you have thick secretions that you'd rather not keep.

Dose and Administration

You can give acetylcysteine via aerosol or apply it topically to the airway (direct instillation). It comes in the following two strengths:

> 20% solution—3 to 5 ml tid or qid
>
> 10% solution—6 to 10 ml tid or qid

Direct instillation of 1 to 2 ml of either of the above is used for patients requiring intubation or placement of an endotracheal tube.

Mode of Action

Acetylcysteine breaks disulfide bonds in mucus, and substitutes its own sulfhydryl groups. The sulfhydryl groups don't bond or cross-link with anything, so both the viscosity and elasticity of mucus decrease. It even works on infected secretions. What a plus!

How long does it take to work? It starts to work on contact!

Q 11. Your patient is about to receive acetylcysteine via SVN. What dose is the best choice? _____

Q 12. Why? _____
_____
_____

Answer: Actually, either 10% or 20% solutions could be used. The amount of milliliters that you put in the SVN will determine how long the treatment will last, so keep it around 6 ml. Direct instillation is only appropriate if the patient's upper airway is bypassed.

Q 13 The worst hazard is bronchospasm, which is more likely to occur in patients with hyperactive airways (like those who have _____).

Minimize this risk by using 10% solution or by giving a bronchodilator with the acetylcysteine.

Q 14 You can also give the bronchodilator first if you don't want to mix them. If you do this, use one with rapid onset and quick peak effect, like _____.

Answer: Isoetharine is the best choice. The more beta-2 specific bronchodilators are too slow!

Also remember that rapid liquefication of secretions can occur once that old acetylcysteine hits them. So if the patient has an artificial airway, you should be ready to suction, just in case.

Acetylcysteine smells horrible because of the release of hydrogen sulfide. This may cause the patient to hurl (vomit).

After three fourths of the solution is nebulized, dilute the rest with an equal amount of sterile water. This prevents airway irritation.

WARNING: Acetylcysteine is incompatible when mixed with the following antibiotics and should *not be combined* in physical solution:

- Sodium ampicillin
- Erythromycin lactobionate
- Amphotericin B
- Tetracyclines

You can give them by different routes of administration. Just don't mix them together physically (like in a solution to be nebulized).

Use with Acetaminophen Overdose

Using acetylcysteine to counteract acetaminophen overdose is an interesting application. In this case, the patient has to drink the acetylcysteine. Acetaminophen (Tylenol) is normally metabolized in the liver. About 4% of it enters a metabolic pathway, and the metabolite that results is toxic to the liver. But the liver has glutathione, which reacts with the metabolite, so there's no harm done. If one overdoses on acetaminophen, there's too much of the toxic metabolite for the glutathione to handle, and it trashes one's liver. I know you're asking, "Why not just give the patient glutathione?" Well, not a bad idea, but it won't cross into the liver cells. Now what to do? Acetylcysteine to the rescue! It's structurally similar to glutathione, and it crosses into the liver, so it takes care of the toxic metabolite and protects the liver. Hooray!

$\mathcal{Q}$15. Acetylcysteine should never be combined with certain _____

$\mathcal{Q}$16. Acetylcysteine can be used to treat _____ overdose.

$\mathcal{Q}$17. Explain in your own words how this works.
_____
_____
_____
_____

Dornase Alfa (Pulmozyme)

Dornase alfa is a clone of the natural human pancreatic DNase enzyme (which digests extracellular DNA—yum). Dornase alfa is an orphan drug. (You've got to look all the way back in Chapter 1 to find out what an orphan drug is if you don't remember!) It is used to treat the really thick secretions in cystic fibrosis.

Dornase alfa breaks down the DNA in the infected secretions. During infection (of which patients with cystic fibrosis get many), neutrophils get together and have a big party in the airway and release DNA. This makes the secretions even thicker. Dornase alfa breaks down the DNA in the infected secretions, and actually lowers the viscosity of the mucus.

$\mathcal{Q}$18. Define viscosity.
_____

$\mathcal{Q}$19. Why is less viscous mucus better for the patient? _____
_____

The catch is that dornase alfa works on infected mucus but not on uninfected mucus. (Uninfected secretions have no DNA.) It can be nebulized in an SVN with an expiratory filter.

Gene Therapy

Another approach to try and normalize airway secretion production in cystic fibrosis has been gene therapy. The abnormal secretions in cystic fibrosis are caused by a genetic mutation; so if a normal copy of the mutated gene is introduced, normal secretory cell function should be the result.

Normal copies of the CFTR gene are being investigated (for direct delivery to the airway) to normalize chloride secretion.

In the United States, the most promising is the adenovirus gene transfer. The adenovirus serves as the taxi, carrying the "good" gene. The subject is infected with the modified virus. The virus infects the airway cells. The normal CFTR gene gets introduced in place of the mutated gene. Normal function begins. They all live happily ever after!

Effect of Bland Aerosols on Mucus

Bland aerosols include distilled water, normal saline (0.9%), and hypertonic and hypotonic saline. Now, remember the Jell-O analogy? *There is no evidence that bland aerosols reduce mucus to a less viscous state by topical hydration or mixing.* Told you so.

Q 20. So why are they used? Even though they don't make mucus less _____, they may sufficiently irritate the airway to stimulate a cough. Hypertonic and hypotonic saline solutions are the most irritating. Are you
irritated by bland people? If you are, this section will be easy for you to remember.

Bland aerosols are basically nothing more than expectorants.

Well, enough talk about mucus. Bring on the NBRC questions!

1. Which of the following represent the two layers/phases of mucus?
   a. Gel and sol
   b. Gel and fal
   c. Sol and fal
   d. a or c   (Chapter 9, p. 154)

2. In surface epithelial cells, which type of cell is predominant?
   a. subepithelial
   b. Clara cells
   c. ciliated cells
   d. goblet cells   (Chapter 9, p. 154)

3. The effect of improving the mobilization and clearance of respiratory secretions is known as which of the following?
   a. Mucoactive
   b. Mucokinetic
   c. Mucolytic
   d. Mucospissic   (Chapter 9, p. 155)

4. All but which of the following slow the rate of mucociliary transport?
   a. Cigarette smoking
   b. Beta agonists
   c. COPD
   d. Hypoxia   (Chapter 9, p. 158)

5. Which of the following classes of drugs does *not* increase mucociliary clearance?
   a. Beta agonists
   b. Xanthines
   c. Corticosteroids
   d. Cholinergics   (Chapter 9, p 158)

6. Which of the following diseases are characterized by mucus hypersecretion?
   I.   Acute bronchitis
   II. Chronic bronchitis
   III. Asthma
   IV. Cystic fibrosis

   a. I, II, III, IV
   b. I, II, III
   c. II, III, IV
   d. I, II, IV   (Chapter 9, pp. 161-162)

7. Which of the following describes the ability of a deformed material to return to its original shape?
   a. Rheoticity
   b. Viscosity
   c. Elasticity
   d. Spinability   (Chapter 9, p. 163)

8. Acetylcysteine is classified as which of the following?
   a. Mucoactive agent
   b. Mucolytic
   c. Mucoviscid
   d. Disulfide   (Chapter 9, p. 165)

9. Acetylcysteine may be delivered by which of the following routes?
   a. Oral
   b. Aerosol
   c. Topical
   d. All the above (Chapter 9, pp. 165-166)

10. Which of the following drugs breaks down the DNA of infected secretions in patients with cystic fibrosis?
    a. Acetylcysteine
    b. Pancreatic dornase
    c. Dornase alfa
    d. Fenoterol   (Chapter 9, p. 167)

Sim

Your patient, Mr. Green, is a 60-year-old white man with chronic bronchitis and mild asthma. His physician, Dr. Pulmo, has asked you to develop a plan for Mr. Green's respiratory care. What elements should you include?

_____

_____

_____

_____

_____

Answer: Prevention (smoking cessation if necessary), avoid pollutants; optimal bronchial hygiene techniques (bronchodilator, hydration, coughing and deep breathing techniques, possibly postural drainage); use of a mucolytic agent; corticosteroids; early recognition and treatment of infection.

Dr. Pulmo okays the bronchodilator and acetylcysteine and education on avoiding pollutants, hydration, cough and deep breathing, and signs and symptoms of infection. Therapy is begun. Mr. Green is less than pleased with the taste and smell of the acetylcysteine, even though it seems to be effective. He asks you how the stuff works. What do you tell him?

_____

_____

_____

Answer: It breaks up the mucus, so that it's not so thick, making it easier for you to cough out. The rotten egg smell is a result of the release of hydrogen sulfide. (He probably doesn't care about the disulfide bonds and sulfhydryl groups, but if he seems to want more info, tell him.)

Because of Mr. Green's asthma, Dr. Pulmo has taken your advice to give a bronchodilator along with the acetylcysteine. Why have you recommended this, and which bronchodilator would you prescribe?

_____

_____

_____

_____

_____

Answer: Bronchospasm is the most serious potential complication associated with acetylcysteine. Use a bronchodilator that is fast acting (or it won't do you any good) (quick onset and peak effect). Isoetharine is a good choice. The bronchodilator may be delivered with the acetylcysteine or before the acetylcysteine treatment.

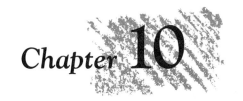

Chapter 10 Surfactant Agents

Surfactants are designed to change the surface tension of airway secretions. Let's define before we go any further:

Surfactant—surface active agent that lowers surface tension; examples are soap and certain kinds of detergents.

Surface tension—a force caused by the attraction between like molecules, which occurs at liquid-gas interfaces, and which holds the liquid surface intact; because liquid molecules are more attracted to each other than they are to gas molecules, they sort of "draw in" on themselves, and a spherical shape is the result. Unit of measure is dyne/cm.

Laplace's Law—Pressure = (4 × Surface tension)/ Radius; this is applied to a drop or bubble, as shown below.

The alveolus has a liquid lining, so surface tension forces apply to it. The higher the surface tension, the greater the compressing force inside the alveolus, which can lead to collapse or difficulty in opening the alveolus.

$\mathcal{Q}$1. On the other hand, the lower the surface tension, the _____ the _____ inside the _____, which makes it _____ to open.

Exogenous Surfactant

Exogenous surfactant is prepared *outside* the patient's own body. You can make it from other humans, animals, or synthetic material. Clinically, exogenous surfactant is used to supply surfactant to the lungs of premature infants because their lungs are immature and don't have enough surfactant (respiratory distress syndrome [RDS]). Exogenous surfactant has also been studied in adult RDS (ARDS). There isn't conclusive evidence yet whether it works.

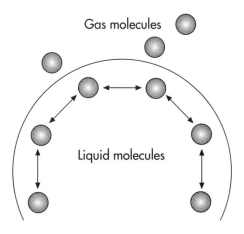

A. Surface tension

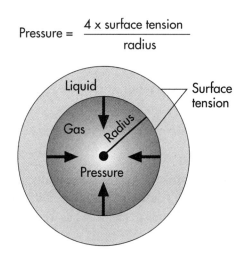

$$\text{Pressure} = \frac{4 \times \text{surface tension}}{\text{radius}}$$

B. Laplace's law

Q2. List three ways to make exogenous surfactant.

1. _____
2. _____
3. _____

Q3. Circle one. In RDS, surface tension is abnormally (high, low).

There are two exogenous surfactant products on the market: colfosceril palmitate (Exosurf) and beractant (Survanta).

Composition of Pulmonary Surfactant

Pulmonary surfactant is made up of lipids (85% to 90%) and proteins (10%). (It's manufactured by type II alveolar cells, and its main function is to regulate surface tension of the liquid lining of the alveolus.)

When you inhale, a stretch response occurs, and these things called lamellar bodies that actually hold the surfactant secrete surfactant into the alveolus. The constant secretion of surfactant is balanced by the following:

Clearance by alveolar macrophages
Endocytosis back into type II cells (recycling)

Actually, 90% to 95% of surfactant is recycled this way.

Q4. Surfactant is secreted by _____ into the _____ .

Q5. So that the lungs aren't overwhelmed by surfactant, most of it is taken back into _____ cells and _____ again.

This is why exogenous surfactant usually only takes one or two doses. It gets taken into the surfactant pool and gets recycled as we just covered.

As a bonus, surfactant enhances ciliary beat frequency and helps maintain airway patency.

Types of Exogenous Surfactant

There are three categories of exogenous surfactant:

1. Natural surfactant is made from animals or humans. You get it by washing out the alveoli or from amniotic fluid.

   The good thing—It's already got the right stuff in it.

   The bad thing(s)—It's expensive and time consuming to get. Plus, you have to worry about contamination.

   You usually add or remove something to get the finished product.

   Different brands are made from minced cow lung, pig lung extract, and alveolar wash from a calf!

2. Synthetic surfactant is made by those clinical types in the lab with no natural ingredients (sounds like gummy bears).

   The good thing—It is free from contamination.

   The bad thing—It doesn't work as well as the natural stuff.

3. Synthetic natural surfactant is the ideal combo, genetically engineered surfactant. It's on the way, expect it in 5 to 10 years.

Q6. Complete the table below.

	Natural Surfactant	Synthetic Surfactant
Advantage		
Disadvantage		

Clinical Application of Exogenous Surfactant

Indications

Indications for clinical application of exogenous surfactant are:

- Prevention of RDS in low birth weight infants
- Prevention of RDS in other infants with immature lungs
- Retroactive (rescue) treatment of infants with RDS

*Q*7. What is the problem with pulmonary surfactant in RDS?

_____

_____

_____

The high surface tensions in those little, immature alveoli require more ventilating pressure to expand (like those little birthday party balloons that drive people crazy). The babies work so hard to inflate their lungs, they tire and ventilatory failure occurs.

Clinical Effect of Exogenous Surfactant

Surfactant's effect is to replace the shallow pool of endogenous surfactant in neonatal RDS. Remember, once it's in the alveolus, it gets recycled. Usually, there's a big improvement in oxygenation after surfactant therapy.

*Q*8. Why do you think this is?

_____

_____

_____

The dose depends on the type and brand used.

Administration

Exogenous surfactant is instilled directly into the endotracheal tube. The method of administration varies somewhat depending on the brand given. Let's look at two types.

1. Colfosceril palmitate (Exosurf) is synthetic. Specifically, the indications for use are the same as the general ones, but with a specific weight of 1350 g (for low birth weight).

   The dose is 5 ml/kg given as two doses. Each vial contains 8 ml of reconstituted (from a powder) suspension.

   If more than one dose is needed, the doses are administered in 12-hour increments.

   Colfosceril palmitate is instilled into the endotracheal tube through a side port, with the infant in the midline position. The dose is given in bursts timed to coincide with inspiration. The baby is rotated to the right and ventilated for 30 seconds. This sequence is repeated on the left.

2. Beractant (Survanta) is a modified natural surfactant (minced cow lung extract).

   It comes in an 8-ml vial (25 mg/ml in a 0.9% sodium chloride solution).

   Beractant's "low birth weight" is defined as 1250 g.

   You don't have to reconstitute beractant because it already comes in suspension.

   Dose is 4 ml/kg given in fourths from a syringe through a 5-F catheter in the endotracheal tube.

   The 5-F catheter is removed, and the baby is manually ventilated for 30 seconds.

   Repeat doses are given no sooner than 6 hours apart.

$\mathcal{Q}$9. Compare colfosceril palmitate (Exosurf) and beractant (Survanta).

Exosurf

_____

_____

_____

_____

Survanta

_____

_____

_____

_____

Hazards and Complications

Because you are delivering relatively large volumes to tiny airways, gas exchange may be blocked, causing desaturation and/or bradycardia.

As a result of surfactant, pulmonary compliance should improve. This may result in the following:

- Overventilation
- Hyperoxygenation with dangerously high PaO_2 levels, which can cause retrolental fibroplasia (RLF) and blindness
- Excessive volume delivery from pressure-limited ventilation

Exogenous surfactant accomplishes the following:

- Improves survival in RDS
- Improves oxygenation
- Reduces the number of days spent on ventilator support
- Reduces the number of days spent on supplemental oxygen

What a great drug! Ready for the questions?

1. Surfactant accomplishes which of the following?
   a. Raises surface tension
   b. Lowers surface tension
   c. Forces molecules to overcome their attraction
   d. b and c   (Chapter 10, p. 177)

2. Which of the following happens as the surface tension of the alveolus' liquid increases?
   a. The easier it is for the alveolus to inflate.
   b. The harder it is for the alveolus to inflate.
   c. The lesser the minute ventilation.
   d. The more type I cells are produced.
                    (Chapter 10, pp. 177-178)

3. Surfactant is produced by which type of alveolar cell?
   a. I
   b. II
   c. III
   d. Macrophage   (Chapter 10, p. 181)

4. Which of the following describes surfactant preparations from outside the patient's body?
   a. Endogenous
   b. Mysogenous
   c. Exogenous
   d. Detergent-type   (Chapter 10, p. 180)

5. Surfactant is composed of which of the following?
   a. A variety of amino acids
   b. 10% lipids and 90% proteins
   c. 50% lipids and 50% proteins
   d. 90% lipids and 10% proteins
                    (Chapter 10, p. 181)

6. Surfactant is constantly secreted into the alveolus. Which of the following mechanisms is most effective in countering this secretion?
   a. The lymphatic system
   b. Alveolar macrophages
   c. Endocytosis into the type II cell
   d. Coughing   (Chapter 10, p. 182)

7. How is natural surfactant obtained?
   a. Cloning
   b. Amniotic fluid
   c. Alveolar wash
   d. b and c   (Chapter 10, p. 183)

8. Which of the following are indications for exogenous surfactant therapy?
   I. Prevention of sudden infant death syndrome in premature infants
   II. Prevention of RDS in low birth weight infants
   III. Rescue treatment for bronchopulmonary hyperplasia
   IV. Rescue treatment for RDS

   a. I, II, III, IV
   b. I, II, III
   c. I and III
   d. II and IV   (Chapter 10, p. 184)

9. How is exogenous surfactant administered?
   a. Aerosol route
   b. Direct instillation into the trachea
   c. IV
   d. Parenteral route
                        (Chapter 10, pp. 185-186)

10. All but which of the following are complications that may occur with the use of exogenous surfactant?
    a. Desaturation
    b. Tachycardia
    c. Hyperoxygenation
    d. Overventilation
                        (Chapter 10, pp.186-187)

Sim

A male infant (30 weeks' gestation) has been transferred to the neonatal ICU, for treatment of impending RDS. The baby weighs 1500 g. Your institution is a university research institution, participating in a multicenter colfosceril palmitate (Exosurf) trial. This baby fits the protocol's inclusion criteria, and the resident asks you to obtain informed consent from the parents. What do you tell them?

_____
_____
_____
_____
_____

Answer: Include the following points in your discussion with the parents. Speak at their level (not over their heads or condescendingly).

Remember, they are frightened and be empathetic and unhurried. Encourage questions so that they can truly make an informed decision.

- The baby's lungs are immature and have not yet manufactured enough surfactant.
- Surfactant makes it easier for the baby to inflate his air sacs (alveoli) because it lowers surface tension.
- The baby is working too hard to breathe. He will tire and require mechanical ventilation until his lungs mature sufficiently.
- The colfosceril palmitate (Exosurf) is artificial surfactant that can be given to the baby to help make breathing easier for him.
- Once he gets the recommended dose, the surfactant will be recycled by his alveoli, and he will probably be extubated sooner. His chance of survival is likely to be better also.

The parents consent to the treatment. What dose will you give after it's reconsituted?

_____

Answer:

The dose is 5 ml/kg $\times$ 1.5 kg (1500 g) = 7.5 ml

How will you administer the colfosceril palmitate (Exosurf)?

_____
_____
_____
_____
_____

Answer:

- Place the baby in midline position
- Give 3.75 ml through the side port adaptor of the endotracheal tube, timed to coincide with inspiration.
- Rotate the baby to the right side and ventilate for 30 seconds.
- Give 3.75 ml (timed to coincide with inspiration) with the baby in midline position.
- Rotate the baby to the left side and ventilate for 30 seconds.
- If the baby does not improve and requires another dose, give the dose in 12 hours.

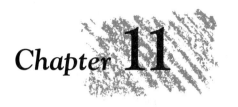

Chapter 11 Corticosteroids in Respiratory Care

Corticosteroids are a group of chemicals secreted by the adrenal cortex. They're adrenal cortical hormones. The adrenal gland has two parts:

1. Inner Zone—produces epinephrine
2. Outer Zone—produces corticosteroids

The corticosteroids used in respiratory care are derivatives of cortisol/hydrocortisone.

The first thing you need to understand is how the body produces and controls its own corticosteroids. The general pathway for release and control of corticosteroids is the hypothalamic-pituitary-adrenal (HPA) axis. (Say that three times, fast!).

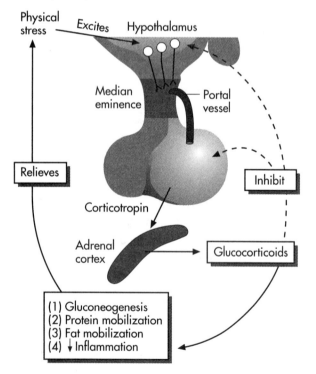

Q 1. Which part of the adrenal gland are we focusing on in this chapter?

_____

Hypothalamic-Pituitary-Adrenal Suppression with Steroid Use

When you treat a patient with exogenous corticosteroids, a side effect (and a big one) is adrenal suppression (HPA suppression).

When the body produces its own (endogenous) glucocorticoids, a feedback mechanism kicks in (within the HPA) to limit production. Danger, Will Robinson!

Your body can't tell the difference between endogenous and exogenous glucocorticoids; so when you give corticosteroids, the same mechanism kicks in, and adrenal production is stalled.

Guess how long it takes for this HPA suppression to happen?

_____

Answer: It takes 24 hours (with systemic administration). Suppression is significant after a week of oral therapy. Are you shocked?

HPA suppression is good reason to use aerosolized corticoster-oids. It minimizes adrenal (HPA) suppression (not to mention fewer side effects and localized treatment).

Q2. Explain HPA suppression in your own words.

_____

_____

_____

_____

_____

The Diurnal Steroid Cycle

Cortisol levels in the body are highest in the morning (around 8 AM). When plasma levels are highest, the HPA suppression mechanism that we talked about kicks in. Plasma levels fall throughout the day. HPA is reactivated to stimulate production of cortisol.

If you give a steroid drug, give it early in the morning when normal tissue levels are high. This way, HPA suppression occurs at the same time it normally would. Then, skip a day to let the body regulate as it's supposed to. This is called (surprise, surprise) alternate day therapy! Side effects are minimized with this approach.

Q3. What would happen if you administered corticosteroids at bedtime? Every day?

_____

_____

_____

_____

Now, on to why we're studying corticosteroids—they reduce inflammation, plain and simple. Asthma is a disease characterized by chronic inflammation of the airway and hyperresponsiveness to various stimuli.

Mast cells and eosinophils are the major players in causing the inflammatory response. The mediators that get released during an asthma attack cause bronchoconstriction, edema, and increased secretions.

The person having the attack experiences wheezing, shortness of breath, tightness in the chest, and cough.

Q4. Treatment with antiinflammatory drugs (like corticosteroids) keeps the basal level of airway inflammation down, so that hyperresponsiveness is _____

_____ .

Your patient has just been prescribed corticosteroids as treatment for his asthma. He is depressed at the thought of having to take yet another drug. Explain to him why this will be a good thing. Practice on a friend. I'll force you to have decent patient education skills if it kills me! You wish.

Are you dying to know exactly how they work? I'll give you the bottom line:

Glucocorticoids inhibit lots of cells that are involved in airway inflammation, like the following:

- Macrophages
- Eosinophils
- Cytokines
- T lymphocytes
- Mast cells

Have you noticed that many of the drugs we've studied have bonus effects? Really, you hadn't noticed? Anyway, a bonus of glucocorticoids is that they also squelch plasma leakage and mucus secretion in those inflamed airways.

Sometimes, in the midst of an asthma attack, the patient is no longer responsive to beta agonists. Another good thing glucocorticoids do is to restore that responsiveness. This can happen 1 to 4 hours after IV administration of glucocorticoids. So if you see a bolus of steroid being administered to an asthmatic patient who is doing poorly, it's being done to restore responsiveness to beta agonists.

Q5. List three great effects that glucocorticoids have going for them.

1. _____

2. _____

3. _____

Drug	Strength	Dose
Dexamethasone sodium phospate (Decadron Respihaler)	84 µg/puff	Adults: 3 puffs tid or qid Children: 2 puffs tid or qid
Beclomethasone dipropionate (Beclovent, Vanceril)	42 µg/puff	Adults: 2 puffs tid or qid Children: 1-2 puffs tid or qid
(Vanceril 84 µg double strength)	84 µg/puff	Adults and children ≥6 yr: bid
Triamcinolone acetonide (Azmacort)	100 µg/puff	Adults: 2 puffs tid or qid Children: 1-2 puffs tid or qid
Flunisolide (AeroBid)	250 µg/puff	Adults: 2 puffs bid Children: 2 puffs bid
Fluticasone propionate (Flovent)	42 µg/puff 110 µg/puff 220 µg/puff	Children >12 yr: 2 puffs bid* 88-220 µg bid, up to 440 µg bid† 880 µg bid‡

*Recommended starting dose if on bronchodilators alone.
†If on inhaled corticosteroids previously.
‡If on oral corticosteroids previously.

Aerosolized Corticosteroids

Remember, systemic corticosteroids have nasty side effects, so geniuses somewhere came up with the idea of aerosolizing them. There are lots to choose from. They're listed in the table above (in chronological order of development, in case you care), along with strength and recommended dose for each.

Some of the steroids available to inhale orally, also come in nasal sprays. These, however, are used to treat nasal conditions, like allergies.

Q 6. Which lasts longer, Decadron or Flovent?

Q 7. How do you know?

Answer: Flovent—It only has to be given bid versus tid or qid for Decadron.

Hazards and Side Effects of Corticosteroids

Side effects associated with systemic administration of corticosteroids include the following:

- HPA suppression
- Immunosuppression
- Osteoporosis
- Fluid retention
- Increased white blood cell count
- Slowing of growth in kids
- Psychiatric reactions
- Cataract formation
- Striated skeletal muscle myopathy
- Hypertension
- Dermatological changes
- Hyperglycemia

Side Effects with Aerosol Administration

Although corticosteroids have far fewer side effects when they're given by aerosol, the following side effects do occur:

Systemic	Local
• HPA suppression • Possible growth • Possible growth slowing in kids	• Oropharyngeal fungal infection • Dysphonia • Cough

The higher the dose (of inhaled corticosteroids), the greater the possibility that the patient will experience side effects.

Also, if you change a patient from systemic to inhaled administration, the patient may experience adrenal insufficiency, extrapulmonary allergy, or acute asthma; so wean the patient gradually from oral to inhaled.

What are some things you could do to minimize the local side effects that occur with inhaled steroid administration?

_____

_____

_____

Answer: Rinse the mouth after administration (to clean out the oropharynx). Use of a spacer also decreases the amount of drug that is deposited in the back of the throat. This will minimize dysphonia and fungal infections. Also, giving the lowest dose possible will minimize the incidence of side effects.

Clinical Application
Because they reduce inflammation, corticosteroids are indicated in the following conditions:

1. Asthma (they're considered *controlling* rather than *relieving* agents)

   - Try inhaled steroids to replace oral steroids.

   - Inhaled steroids plus beta agonists reduce morbidity and airway hyperresponsiveness.

   - Because of the growth-slowing aspect, try cromolyn sodium first where kids are concerned.

Other points to be recognized include the following:

1. Don't use a corticosteroid to treat an acute asthma attack. Systemic application is indicated here.

   𝒬8. Remember why? _____

   _____

2. Always use a spacer device.

𝒬9. Remember why? _____

_____

3. Treatment of related bronchospastic states is not controlled by other therapy.

4. Corticosteroids may be used to control seasonal allergic or nonallergic rhinitis.

Use of Corticosteroids in Chronic Obstructive Pulmonary Disease
Could it be true? It's debatable—ipratropium is the drug of choice, though.

𝒬10. What class of bronchodilator is ipratropium?

_____

Don't you hate it when ancient history is rehashed?

P.S. Corticosteroids are different from anabolic steroids—you know, the stuff all the guys and gals in big-time wrestling are so fond of.

Go crazy

1. Corticosteroids are naturally secreted by which of the following?
   a. Thymal cortex—outer zone
   b. Adrenal cortex—outer zone
   c. Adrenal cortex—inner zone
   d. Thymal cortex—inner zone
      (Chapter 11, p. 191)

2. Optimally, exogenous glucocorticoids should be taken when?
   a. Early in the morning
   b. With milk
   c. At bedtime
   d. On an empty stomach
      (Chapter 11, p. 193)

3. Corticosteroids are described as which of the following?
   a. Bronchodilators
   b. Smooth muscle dilators
   c. Antiinflammatory
   d. Lipid soluble   (Chapter 11, p. 191)

4. Which of the following occur during an asthma attack?
   - I. Bronchospasm
   - II. Release of epinephrine
   - III. Mucosal edema
   - IV. Increased secretions

   a. I, II, III, IV
   b. I, II, III
   c. I, III, IV
   d. II, III, IV   (Chapter 11, p. 195)

5. Glucocorticoids inhibit all but which of the following?
   a. Ectokines
   b. Macrophages
   c. Lymphocytes
   d. Mast cells   (Chapter 11, p. 197)

6. Which of the following represents an advantage of local over systemic administration of corticosteroids?
   a. Greater systemic side effects
   b. Higher dose required
   c. Direct acting
   d. No side effects
                (Chapter 11, pp. 198-199)

7. Allergic and nonallergic rhinitis would be treated with which of the following forms of corticosteroid?
   a. Pill
   b. Nasal spray
   c. Aerosol
   d. Injection   (Chapter 11, p. 201)

8. All but which of the following are side effects seen with systemic administration of corticosteroids?
   a. HPA suppression
   b. Growth retardation
   c. Diuresis
   d. Osteoporosis   (Chapter 11, p. 202)

9. Which of the following describes aerosol administration of corticosteroids:
   a. Is associated with no side effects
   b. Produces severe side effects
   c. Results in more systemic than local side effects
   d. Results in more local than systemic side effects   (Chapter 11, p. 203)

10. Which of the following minimizes local side effects associated with use of inhaled corticosteroids?
    a. Use a spacer device
    b. Rinse mouth after each treatment
    c. Prescribe the lowest dose possible
    d. All the above   (Chapter 11, p. 204)

Sim

Mrs. Peacock (can you tell I played too much Clue as a child?) has been prescribed triamcinolone (Azmacort) 100 µg/puff (2 puffs qid), as treatment for moderate asthma. How much triamcinolone will she receive in a 24-hour period?

_____

Answer: 100 µg/puff $\times$ 2 = 200 µg/treament $\times$ 4 = 800 µg/day

When instructing her in the use of her MDI, what must you include?

_____
_____
_____
_____
_____

Answer: Make sure that Mrs. Peacock can demonstrate proper MDI technique. (If you forget what this is, go back to Chapter 3.) Stress the importance of using a spacer device so that less of the drug is deposited in the back of her throat, so she's less likely to get a fungal infection; stress rinsing her mouth out and/or gargling after each treatment, also to minimize her chances of fungal infection. Let her know that she may also experience dysphonia (hoarseness or change in voice quality), cough, or mild bronchospasm, and that if she does, she should notify you to contact her physician and discuss other options. These would include other corticosteroids or a lower dose of triamcinolone. What a good and concerned therapist you are.

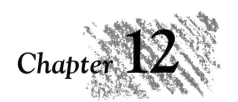

Chapter 12 Mediator Antagonists

In this chapter we'll take a look at drugs that inhibit inflammatory cells (like mast cells) and/or act as antagonists to mediators of inflammation.

INFLAMMATION IN ASTHMA

Asthma is a chronic inflammatory disease of the airways. It can be either extrinsic (triggered by an allergy) or intrinsic (not associated with sensitization to inhaled allergens). Extrinsic is more common in kids; intrinsic is more common in adults.

In both types of asthma, mediators (like histamine) and enzymes are released and act on target tissue in the airway. Plus, inflammatory cells are recruited and activated in the airway.

Q1. The result is bronchoconstriction, mucus secretion, and mucosal edema. All these things combine to cause airway obstruction and _____ flow rates.

Q2. Compare and contrast extrinsic and intrinsic asthma.

Extrinsic   **Intrinsic**

_____   _____
_____   _____
_____   _____
_____   _____

If all that wasn't enough, T lymphocytes release cytokines, which cause accumulation and activation of eosinophils. Chemicals are released by

the eosinophils. Further airway damage (increased inflammation) occurs.

Q3. List four things that cause airway narrowing during an asthma attack.
1. _____
2. _____
3. _____
4. _____

This chapter focuses on drugs that inhibit inflammatory mediators/cells in an effort to control the asthmatic response.

Cromolyn Sodium (Disodium Chromoglycate)

Cromolyn sodium has been around since 1973. It's a prophylactic to prevent asthma reactions.

It's *not* related to a bronchodilator or a corticosteroid.

Q4. Hey, go ahead and list the three classes of bronchodilators, just for fun. (Hint: Chapters 6, 7, and 8.)
1. _____
2. _____
3. _____

Indications

- Prophylactic management of bronchial asthma (as opposed to what—cranial asthma?)
- Prevention of exercise-induced bronchospasm (EIB)
- Allergic rhinitis (nasal solution)

Mode of Action

Hurry—hurry—hurry! It's not just an antiasth-matic! It's an antiallergic! It's a mast cell stabi-lizer!

But seriously, cromolyn sodium stabilizes mast cells, preventing the release of histamine, so that the whole nasty sequence of events never takes place. (Histamine is the bad seed.) And (can you believe your luck?), no one's really sure just how this all happens!

*Q*5. When mast cells degranulate, histamine is released, causing _____, _____, and _____.

So, how do you deliver cromolyn sodium? For the asthma-type indications, you've got your choice of the following three delivery devices:

1. DPI (Spinhaler)—20 mg
2. SVN—20 mg in 2 ml of solution
3. MDI—2 mg

*Q*6. Think back—back—to Chapter 3. For a patient to be able to use a DPI, what criteria must the patient meet?
   a. Able to perform breath-hold
   b. Able to generate high inspiratory flow rates
   c. Able to follow instructions
   d. All the above

Side Effects
Really, cromolyn sodium is pretty safe. Only 2% of patients experience side effects, and these side effects aren't that bad.

With DPI:

- Throat irritation
- Dry mouth
- Wheezing
- Hoarseness
- Cough

What can you do to minimize these? Try a beta agonist or switch to MDI or SVN.

With SVN:

- Cough
- Wheezing
- Nasal itching
- Nasal congestion
- Sneezing

How many patients experience side effects with cromolyn sodium use? _____ %

Answer: Only 2! Pretty good odds unless you're one of that 2%.

Clinical Efficacy
Cromolyn sodium works in about 70% of patients.

Clinical Application
Cromolyn sodium is a prophylactic. (*Don't use it during an asthma attack!*)

Write the following three times: Don't use cro-molyn sodium during an acute asthma attack!

_____

_____

_____

Once the histamine has been released, mast cell stabilization is not an option and may even cause further airway irritation.

- It may take 2 to 4 weeks for the patient's symptoms to improve.
- You can't just take a patient off cortico-steroids and switch the patient to cromolyn sodium. Don't forget HPA suppression! Remember, you've got to wean the patient off slowly.

Guidelines for the management of asthma say that cromolyn sodium should be used in patients who already get beta agonists for control of their asthma. It's basically used as an alternative to inhaled corticosteroids in kids.

*Q*7. Why are steroids bad (or potentially bad) for kids?

_____

Dosage Regulation

For seasonal allergy treatment, start therapy about a week before allergen exposure.
For EIB, give it 15 minutes before exercise.

For allergen exposure (like if you have to have lunch with Aunt Matilda and her cats, and you're allergic to cat hair), take it 30 minutes before exposure.

Nedocromil Sodium (Tilade)

Nedocromil sodium has only been around since 1992. It's also an inhaled prophylactic antiasthmatic. It's similar to cromolyn sodium in its action and clinical application, so this section should be almost a review for cromolyn as well.

Indications
- Prophylactic drug for treatment of mild to moderate asthma

  ℚ8. Remember, it's a controller, not a reliever, so *never* use it during

  _____.

Dosage and Administration
- MDI 2 puffs qid (1.75 mg/puff)

Mode of Action
- Inhibits inflammatory cells, including mast cells and eosinophils

Side Effects
Hardly any, but the most common are:

- Unpleasant taste
- Nausea/vomiting
- Headache
- Dizziness

Clinical Efficacy
For adults—Improvement was greatest in mild to moderate asthma and when used with bronchodilator therapy.

For kids—There seems to be significant improvement in peak flow rates and a decrease in use of bronchodilators. As a bonus, 4 mg bid has been shown to be as effective as 5 mg cromolyn sodium qid.

ℚ9. What is the implication of prescribing less medicine less often?

_____

_____

_____

Zafirlukast (Accolate)

Now comes a new drug, zafirlukast (Accolate), only approved for use in the United States in late 1996. Is this the cutting edge, or what? It's indicated for the prophylactic and long-term treatment of asthma, approved for use in people older than 12 years, and taken as a tablet (20 mg bid) or inhaled (200 mg).

Mode of Action
It acts on leukotrienes, preventing the inflammatory response of airway contractility, vascular permeability, and mucus secretion.

It works on asthma reactions caused by exercise, cold air, allergens, and aspirin (intrinsic).

The oral form offers more advantages than the inhaled form:

- More rapid absorption
- Inhibits both early and late phases of asthma (Inhaled form inhibits only early phase.)
- Also causes bronchodilation

Side Effects
- Headache
- Nausea
- Generalized and abdominal pain
- Infection (mostly respiratory)
- Diarrhea

Clinical Application
- Prevention of bronchoconstriction— alternative to inhaled corticosteroids in mild persistent asthma in subjects older than 12 years

Zileuton

If you thought zafirlukast was new, stand back! Zileuton was approved for use in early 1997. It's indicated for the prophylaxis and long-term treatment of asthma.

It's available as a 600-mg tablet, taken bid, and is approved for use in the over 12 set.

*Q*10. Like the other drugs in this chapter, zileuton is a _____, not a reliever, so don't ever use it during _____.

Mode of Action
Zileuton (sounds like a *Star Wars* character) interrupts the synthesis of leukotrienes so that they can't contribute to the inflammatory response.

Hazards and Side Effects
- Headache
- Abdominal pain
- General pain
- Dyspepsia
- Loss of strength (don't prescribe it for Hercules)
- Some liver function test values have been elevated with use of zileuton, so monitor this. Symptoms of liver dysfunction include the following:
  - Right upper quadrant pain
  - Flu-like symptoms
  - Jaundice
  - Nausea
  - Fatigue

*Q*11. Compare and contrast zafirlukast and zileuton.

Zafirlukast	Zileuton
_____	_____
_____	_____
_____	_____
_____	_____

On to the questions!

1. If a patient experiences an asthma attack as a result of exposure to cats, the asthma would be categorized as which of the following?
   a. Intrinsic
   b. Extrinsic
   c. Autoimmune
   d. Intangible   (Chapter 12, p. 211)

2. All but which of the following occurs during as asthma attack?
   a. Bronchospasm
   b. Mucosal edema
   c. Increased secretion production
   d. Cilial hyperactivity
                    (Chapter 12, p. 212)

3. Cytokines accomplish which of the following?
   a. Are released by B lymphocytes
   b. Cause sloughing and death of eosinophils
   c. Cause accumulation of eosinophils
   d. a and b   (Chapter 12, p. 212)

4. The increase and activation of eosinophils are associated with which of the following?
   a. Preasthma attack
   b. Increased airway inflammation
   c. Lessened asthma severity
   d. Decreased production of leukotrienes
                    (Chapter 12, pp. 212-213)

5. Cromolyn sodium is classified as which of the following:
   a. Bronchodilator
   b. Cholinergic
   c. Corticosteroid
   d. Antiasthmatic   (Chapter 12, p. 214)

6. Cromolyn sodium is indicated in all but which of the following conditions?
   a. Acute asthma
   b. Asthma prophylaxis
   c. EIB
   d. Allergic rhinitis   (Chapter 12, p. 215)

7. Cromolyn sodium accomplishes which of the following?
   I.   Stabilizes leukotrienes
   II. Stabilizes mast cells
   III. Prevents histamine release
   IV. Prevents eosinophil degranulation

   a. I and III
   b. I and IV
   c. II and III
   d. II and IV   (Chapter 12, p. 215)

8. Cromolyn sodium is available for use in all but which of the following delivery devices?
   a. SPAG
   b. SVN
   c. MDI
   d. DPI   (Chapter 12, p. 217)

9. Which of the following represents the incidence of side effects occurring with cromolyn sodium use?
   a. 20%
   b. 10%
   c. 2%
   d. None reported   (Chapter 12, p. 218)

10. Which of the following describes antiasthmatic drugs?
    a. Tolerance-producing
    b. Symptomatic
    c. Relievers
    d. Controllers   (Chapter 12, p. 219)

Sim

Your patient, Bruce Jenkins, is a world class decathlete who suffers from EIB. His physician has prescribed a beta agonist to treat his bronchospasm and has asked for your recommendation as to which antiasthmatic to try on Bruce. What do you recommend?

_____

Why?

_____

_____

Answer: Try cromolyn sodium first. It's been proven to be effective in EIB, and it's been around the longest, so more is known about its effects (side, clinical).

How much should he take, using which delivery device?

_____

_____

Answer: Bruce can understand and follow directions, perform inspiratory hold, and generate enough flow for DPI, so nothing precludes him from any of the delivery devices available. Therefore delivery device is a matter of personal preference. Certainly, MDI is probably the most commonly prescribed, uses the lowest dose, and is convenient and easy to use. If this is the method you selected, Bruce should take 2 puffs (2 mg), 15 minutes before exercising.

Bruce forgets his meds before exercise one day and experiences bronchospasm. What should he do?

_____

_____

Answer: If you said that he should go home and get his cromolyn sodium MDI, just burn your book and quit respiratory school! Remember, never, _never_ treat bronchospasm with an antiasthmatic. The purpose of antiasthmatics is to prevent inflammation. Once the inflammation and bronchospasm have occurred, you need a beta agonist. Caution Mr. Jenkins that he should never exercise without taking his MDIs wherever he goes.

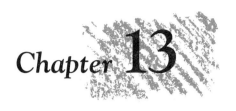

Chapter 13   Aerosolized Antiinfective Agents

Two antiinfective drugs are approved for aerosol administration: pentamidine isethionate (NebuPent) and ribavirin (Virazole). Pentamidine is used to treat *Pneumocystis carinii* pneumonia (PCP) in patients with AIDS. Ribavirin is used for treating respiratory syncytial virus (RSV).

A variety of antibiotics have been aerosolized to treat respiratory infections like cystic fibrosis.

Aerosolized Pentamidine

Pentamidine isethionate is an antiprotozoal that is active against *P. carinii*, which causes PCP. It can be given parenterally (IV or IM) or by aerosol. When it's given parenterally, the drug binds to tissues in the major organs and is stored there sometimes for as long as 9 months—not good. We are all infected with *P. carinii* by the time we're 2 years old. Disease only occurs if the immune system is suppressed.

Indications
Okay, aerosolized pentamidine is used to treat PCP, but more specific indications are as follows:

- A history of one or more episodes of PCP
- CD4+ lymphocyte count of less than or equal to 200/mm^3

It's used to both prevent and treat PCP.

Why Use An Aerosol?
- PCP is located in the alveoli. Inhaled administration targets the lung!
- Parenteral administration has nasty and numerous side effects.
- Aerosolized pentamidine produces higher concentrations in the lung than does IV administration.

*Q*1. What is one bad thing that can happen with IV administration?

_____

_____

Mode of Action
Who knows? It blocks DNA and RNA synthesis.

Side Effects of Parenteral Administration
More than 50% of patients experience adverse effects, like the following:

- IM—pain, swelling, and abscess formation at injection site
- IV—thrombophlebitis
- Hypoglycemia
- Impaired renal function
- Hypotension
- Leukopenia
- Hepatic dysfunction

Side Effects of Aerosol Administration
Side effects can be divided into local and systemic effects:

Local	Systemic
• Cough/bronchial irritation	• Conjunctivitis
• Dyspnea	• Rash
• Bad taste	• Neutropenia
• Wheezing/ bronchospasm (11%)	• Renal insufficiency
• Spontaneous pneumothoraces	• Hypoglycemia/ diabetes
	• Appearance of extrapulmonary *P. carinii* infection

*Q*2. Which side effects occur with both aerosol and parenteral administration?

_____

_____

_____

When patients receive long-term aerosol treatment, the drug accumulates in tissue just like with parenteral administration, producing the same side effects.

*Q*3. How could you prevent the airway effects? _____

_____

_____

Right! What would we do without bronchodilators? Both beta-adrenergic and anticholinergic drugs have been shown to be effective.

Administration of Aerosolized Pentamidine

Dose

For prophylaxis of PCP give 300 mg, once q4wk. Pentamidine (NebuPent) is a dry powder (300 mg) that must be reconstituted in 6 ml of sterile water.

Administration

Use the Respirgard II nebulizer. It's an SVN with a series of one-way valves and an expiratory filter. Here's what it looks like:

It should be powered by 50 psi (duh) at a flow rate of 5 to 7 L/min (just like other SVNs). There are other similar nebs, called the AeroTech II, Fisoneb, and Pulmasonic. (Who comes up with these names anyway?) The only one officially approved by the FDA is the old Respirgard II!

Health care workers have experienced conjunctivitis and bronchospasm as a result of exposure to pentamidine, so the following list should help reduce the amount of drug exposure, as well as TB infection (which is often associated with HIV-positive patients).

1. Stop nebulization if the patient removes the mouthpiece. If the neb has a thumb port, this is easy to do.
2. Use SVNs with one-way valves and an expiratory filter.
3. Use SVNs that produce particles of 1 to 2 μm to ensure maximal airway deposition.
4. Screen patients for cough history and pretreat with a beta agonist if necessary.
5. Give the treatment in a negative pressure room or isolation booth.
6. Use universal precautions.
7. Screen HIV-positive patients for TB.
8. Pregnant and nursing health care workers should avoid exposure to the drug.

Review the above list.

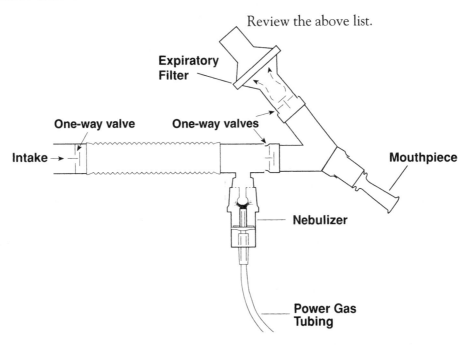

$\mathcal{Q}$4. Which are the easiest to do?

_____

_____

$\mathcal{Q}$5. Which may not be feasible?

_____

_____

There is a drug called TMP-SMX. (You don't need to know what all the letters stand for, unless you're extremely anal-retentive!) TMP-SMX has been shown to be more effective in preventing PCP than pentamidine, as long as the patient can tolerate the side effects. It's what the Centers for Disease Control and Prevention (CDC) recommends for prophylactic therapy.

RIBAVIRIN (Virazole)

Ribavirin is an antiviral, active against the following:

- RSV
- Influenza
- Herpes simplex

It's virostatic, not virucidal, so it only inhibits DNA and RNA viruses. When it's given by aerosol, drug levels are greater in the sputum than in the blood stream.

Indications
Ribavirin is indicated for the following:

- Hospitalized infants and young children with severe lower respiratory tract infections caused by RSV, which will result in bronchiolitis or pneumonia
- All patients receiving mechanical ventilation because of RSV
- Infants and children at serious risk for developing severe lower respiratory tract disease.

Nature of Viral Infection
What's a virus? It is an obligate intracellular parasite containing RNA or DNA, which reproduces by synthesis of subunits within the host cell and causes disease as a result of this replication. Take a look at the drawings below. The first is the structure of a virus; the second shows the concept and sequence of viral infection.

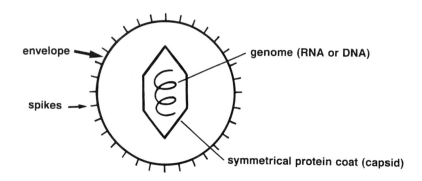

Virion: extracellular virus particle

In the second figure you can see that the virus attaches to the cell (stinking intracellular parasite that it is!), penetrates, uncoats (!), recodes the DNA of the cell, replicates, and leaves the cell. Sort of like Austin Powers, International Man of Mystery!

The host may die in the process. Clinically, no signs occur until the virus leaves the cell (the initial latent period). Sneaky.

$\mathcal{Q}$6. Try to think of three places that you could screw up that sequence of events. (Foil the spy, like a counterspy or something. I told you I played too much Clue.)

1. _____

2. _____

3. _____

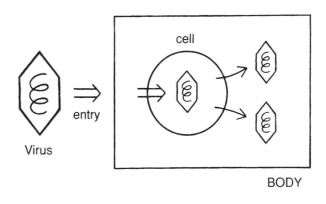

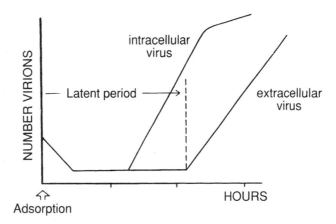

The answers are listed below. If you got only one correct, you are a traitor to your virus; two correct, you are a Virus Bond apprentice; all three, Virus Bond!

1. Prevent the intracellular virus from entering the cell.

2. Prevent the virus from replicating.

3. Prevent the virus from leaving the cell.

RSV can cause bronchiolitis and pneumonia. Most kids get exposed to it by the age of 2 and are not terribly bothered by it. Outbreaks are seasonal, peaking in the winter. (Your mother was right!) RSV spreads by personal contact or hand contamination from surfaces, and there isn't a vaccine.

Mode of Action

Who knows? I love that.

Side Effects

Pulmonary—worsening pulmonary function; pneumothorax; apnea; bacterial pneumonia

Cardiovascular—instability (hypotension, cardiac arrest, digitalis toxicity)

Dermatological/topical—rash; conjunctivitis; eyelid erythema

Equipment-related—occlusion of expiratory valves and sensors with ventilator use; endotracheal tube blockage from drug precipitate

Guess which one is the most common.

Answer: Worsening pulmonary function.

Dose and Administration

Ribavirin should be given in a 20-mg/ml solution, administered by SPAG-2 for 12 to 18 hr/day for 3 to 7 days. You get the drug as 6 g of

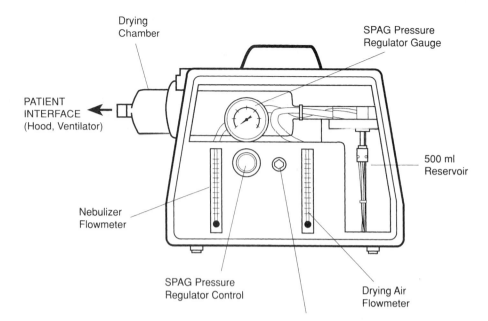

Drying Chamber

SPAG Pressure Regulator Gauge

PATIENT INTERFACE (Hood, Ventilator)

500 ml Reservoir

Nebulizer Flowmeter

SPAG Pressure Regulator Control

Drying Air Flowmeter

powder in a 100-ml vial. You've got to reconstitute it and dilute it to get the correct concentration.

There's a drawing of the SPAG above.

Treatment with ribavirin via the SPAG has been shown to decrease the duration of ventilation, oxygen support, and hospital stay. You junior administrators will like that!

Environmental Contamination
Ribavirin is teratogenic (kills the embryo) in animal species, so pregnant patients and health care workers should steer clear of it. Side effects reported by health care workers include precipitation on contact lenses and conjunctivitis. The drug should be given in well-ventilated areas (at least 6 air changes per hour).

Should you administer ribavirin if you are trying to become pregnant but aren't yet?

_____

Answer: Not if you can avoid it.

Clinical Application
Ribavirin is expensive. The junior administrators will not like that. Plus, there's the environmental exposure concern. The jury is out as to whether this drug is really effective in high-risk patients.

Respiratory Syncytial Virus Immune Globulin Intravenous (Human)

What is RSV immune globulin intravenous? It's a specific antibody to RSV (passive immunity) recently approved by the FDA (early 1996). It's RSV-IGIV, available as Respigam.

Indications
RSV-IGIV is indicated to prevent serious lower respiratory tract infections in kids younger than 2 years with bronchopulmonary dysplasia (BPD) or a history of premature birth (<35 weeks' gestation).

Q7. Give two different examples of kids who could get RSV-IGIV.
   1. _____
   2. _____

Q8. The RSV-IGIV is delivered via _____. What do you think the IV stands for!?

Adverse Reactions
- Fluid overload
- Fever
- Dyspnea
- Myalgia
- Dizziness
- Palpitations
- Abdominal cramps
- Change in blood pressure

You can control these pretty well with the rate of infusion.

Aerosolized Antibiotics

Why aerosolized antibiotics? You can deliver the drug to the target organ with fewer systemic side effects. This delivery route is used to treat gram-negative and fungal pulmonary infections.

Use in Cystic Fibrosis

Patients with cystic fibrosis often come down with gram-negative infections caused by *Pseudomonas aeruginosa*, *Haemophilus influenzae*, *Pseudomonas cepacia*, not to mention *Staphylococcus aureus* (gram positive).

When aerosolized, gentamicin and tobramycin work well in treating such infections. Gentamicin is a tad thick, so you should use a flow rate of 10 to 12 L/min when giving it. The aerosolized route of administration is better than IV for these patients because of the following:

- Lung levels of gentamicin and tobramycin are greater
- Less expensive
- Easier to use at home

Indications for aerosolized antibiotic therapy in cystic fibrosis include the following:

- To maintain present lung function or reduce the rate of deterioration
- To treat or prevent early colonization with *P. aeruginosa*
- To treat acute episodes of respiratory infections

*Q*9. What flow rate should you use to deliver gentamicin via aerosol?

_____

*Q*10. Tobramycin? _____

Side Effects

*Q*11. To prevent local airway irritation when using aerosolized antibiotics, you may need to pretreat with a _____.

Let's go to the NBRC questions.

1. Pentamidine is considered to be which of the following?
   a. Antifungal
   b. Antiparasitic
   c. Antiprotozoal
   d. Antibacterial   (Chapter 13, p. 228)

2. Pentamidine may be administered via which of the following route(s) of administration?
   a. Oral
   b. Inhalation
   c. IV
   d. b and c   (Chapter 13, p. 231)

3. Which route of pentamidine administration is associated with the fewest side effects?
   a. Oral
   b. Inhalation
   c. IV
   d. IM   (Chapter 13, p. 231)

4. Pentamidine for the prophylactic treatment of PCP in HIV-positive patients is administered how frequently?
   a. bid
   b. qid
   c. Weekly
   d. q4wk   (Chapter 13, p. 234)

5. The only device currently approved by the FDA for the administration of pentamidine (NebuPent) is which of the following:
   a. SPAG-2
   b. Respirgard II
   c. AeroTech II
   d. Fisoneb   (Chapter 13, p. 231)

6. SVNs used to deliver pentamidine should be equipped with which of the following?
   I. Inspiratory filter
   II. Expiratory filter
   III. One-way valves
   IV. Compression generators

   a. I, I, III, IV
   b. II and III
   c. I and II
   d. I, II, IV   (Chapter 13, pp. 232-233)

7. Ribavirin is classified as which of the following?
   a. Antiprotozoal
   b. Antifungal
   c. Antibacterial
   d. Antiviral   (Chapter 13, p. 234)

8. Which of the following describes ribavirin (Virazole)?
   a. Virostatic
   b. Virucidal
   c. Bacteriostatic
   d. Bactericidal   (Chapter 13, p. 234)

9. Signs of a viral infection occur when?
   a. Before the initial latent period
   b. After the initial latent period
   c. As the virus is replicating
   d. As the virus uncoats
      (Chapter 13, p. 235)

10. RSV-IGIV is used to prevent serious lower respiratory tract infection with RSV in which patient population?
    a. Children younger than 24 months
    b. Children older than 24 months
    c. Children younger than 24 months with a history of premature birth
    d. Children older than 24 months with cystic fibrosis   (Chapter 13, p. 240)

Sim

Your patient, who has been HIV positive since 1994, presents with a CD4+ count of 100/mm³, fever, shaking chills, and productive cough. He has had PCP once prior to this admission. His diagnosis is PCP, and his physician has ordered pentamidine isethionate (NebuPent) treatments qid to treat it. As you do your pretreatment assessment, the patient tells you that he has previously been given pentamidine and that it makes him cough uncontrollably. What do you recommend?

_____

_____

Answer: Pretreatment with a bronchodilator!

As a favor to you (you're soooo busy), one of your colleagues begins this treatment using an SVN. What's wrong with this picture?

_____

_____

_____

Answer: Pentamidine should be delivered using a Respirgard II, which comes complete with expiratory filter and one-way valves at no extra charge. Well, maybe there is an extra charge, who knows?

Other than using the Respirgard II, what precautions should you take to minimize your exposure to the pentamidine?

_____

_____

_____

Answer: Stop nebulization if the patient removes the mouthpiece; screen patient for TB; avoid exposure if you're pregnant or nursing; administer the treatment in a room with at least six air changes per hour; use universal precautions.

What adverse effects are you likeliest to suffer as a result of exposure to pentamidine?

_____

_____

Answer: Conjunctivitis and bronchospasm.

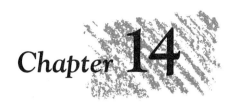# Chapter 14 Antiinfective Agents

You'll see lots of infections if you stick with respiratory care—something to look forward to—pneumonias, acute and chronic bronchitis, bronchiectasis, TB, etc., caused by bacteria, fungus, viruses, and protozoa. This chapter focuses on antibiotic and antiinfective drugs to treat those infections. Before we start, let's differentiate between antibiotic and antiinfective.

Antibiotic—substance produced by microorganisms capable of inhibiting or killing bacteria and other microorganisms

Antiinfective—broader term; includes chemicals that are toxic to bacteria and other microorganisms but are not produced by or derived from those organisms

Modes of Action of Antibiotics

Antibiotics can use the following kill tactics against microorganisms:

1. Inhibition of cell wall synthesis—Bacteria have rigid cell walls. (They need it to protect themselves.) Without the cell wall, the high osmotic pressure will make the cell explode! This is my personal favorite! Antibiotics that do this include penicillin, cephalosporins, vancomycin, and bacitracin.

2. Alteration of cell membrane permeability—This upsets the necessary flow and storage of cell material required for growth and life. Bad news for the bacteria. Antibiotics that like this approach are polymyxins.

3. Inhibition of protein synthesis—Protein synthesis is necessary to a cell's growth and function. Lots of antibiotics interfere with the ribosome's ability to synthesize necessary proteins. Chloramphenicol, tetracyclines, erythromycin, streptomycin, and gentamicin use this tactic.

4. Inhibition of nucleic acid synthesis—DNA synthesis is necessary for life. It's the master code for cell function and activity. Certain antibiotics (like sulfonamides and rifampin) attach to DNA strands and block the DNA replication.

*Q*1. What's the difference between antibiotic and antiinfective?

_____

_____

Here are a few more definitions. (You can never get too many!)

Bacteriostatic—drug that inhibits the growth of a microorganism

Bactericidal—drug that kills a microorganism

Examples of bacteriostatic and bactericidal drugs are listed below.

Bactericidal Antimicrobials	Bacteriostatic Antimicrobials
Penicillins	Chloramphenicol
Cephalosporins	Erythromycin
Cycloserine	Tetracyclines
Vancomycin	Lincomycin
Vacitracin	Sulfonamides
Aminoglycosides	
Polymyxins	

Broad spectrum—useful against a wide range of organisms, both gram-positive and gram-negative bacteria

Narrow spectrum—useful against only a few organisms

Examples of broad- and narrow-spectrum antibiotics are listed below.

Broad	Narrow
Chloramphenicol	Penicillin
Tetracyclines	Streptomycin
Kanamycin	Erythromycin
Cephalosporins	Lincomycin
Ampicillin	Polymyxin B
	Vancomycin

Defense Mechanisms of Antibiotics

Lest you think the bacteria just lie down and take the assault of modern medicine, here are some of the nasty little things they do to survive. You've heard of those drug-resistant strains we get when people don't finish their prescription. It gets much worse.

1. Some bacteria produce an enzyme—penicillinase or beta-lactamase—that can inactivate an antibiotic. *Haemophilus influenzae* and *Staphylococcus aureus* are examples.

2. *Streptococcus pneumoniae* have the ability to put up fake walls, so that antibiotics can't destroy them. (Remember how some antibiotics work by reinventing bacterial cell wall synthesis?)

3. Certain antibiotics enter bacteria through water-filled channels, called porins. Some clever bacteria (like *Pseudomonas aeruginosa*) change the porin protein composition so that the antibiotic entrance is either slowed or prevented altogether.

4. *P. aeruginosa*, *Proteus vulgaris* (you've gotta love that name!), and *S. aureus* actually have pumps to actively remove the antibiotics before they can bind to the target organs—kind of like bouncers.

Q2. Choose your favorite bacteria and explain their defense mechanism.

_____

_____

Now, we'll briefly cover the types of antibiotics and how they work.

BETA-LACTAM ANTIBIOTICS

There are four types of beta-lactam antibiotics. All are bactericidal, acting by messing with bacterial wall synthesis.

Q3. By the way, which organism would mount a defense to this approach?

_____

Penicillin

Penicillin includes natural penicillin (PCN G), penicillinase-resistant agents (methicillin, oxacillin), and broad-spectrum penicillin (ampicillin, carbenicillin).

They act by inhibiting bacterial wall synthesis by inhibiting transpeptidation reactions necessary for cell wall structure.

Bacteria that are resistant to penicillin include the ones that produce penicillinase.

Q4. What is penicillinase and how does it work against penicillin?

_____

_____

Allergy to penicillin is more common with parenteral versus oral administration. Symptoms range from skin rash to anaphylactic shock.

Penicillin is used to treat streptococcal species, *H. influenzae*, and gonococcal and syphilis-causing organisms.

Cephalosporins

Cephalosporins were originally derived from a fungus—yuk! Cephalosporins are used to treat gram-positive organisms (pneumococci, strepto-cocci, staphylococci) and gram-negative ones (*H. influenzae*, *Enterobacter*, *Klebsiella*). None work against *P. aeruginosa*. Pity.

*Q*5. Cephalosporins work by inhibiting bacterial wall synthesis, the same as _____. They're used because they're effective against a lot of common bacteria.

Side effects include nephrotoxicity (I hate when that happens), thrombophlebitis, and pain at the injection site (IM).

Carbapenems

Carbapenems are broad-spectrum antibiotics, effective against many gram-positive and gram-negative organisms. There are only two: Primaxin and Merrem IV.

*Q*6. Carbapenems act by _____ _____. Remember, they're part of the beta-lactam group.

Monobactam

The only drug in the monobactam group is Azactam. It works against many gram-negative aerobic organisms.

*Q*7. If you had a patient with a gram-positive pneumonia, which drugs in the beta-lactam group would be feasible choices?

_____
_____
_____

*Q*8. What about infection with *Klebsiella*? (It's gram negative.)

_____
_____

Aminoglycosides

Aminoglycosides are derived from different species of *Streptomyces*. They work by preventing and distorting bacterial wall synthesis.

Aminoglycosides are used to treat gram-negative pneumonias except for infection with *H. influenzae*, for which gentamicin and tobramycin are used.

Aminoglycosides are commonly aerosolized to treat *Pseudomonas* infection in cystic fibrosis. Streptomycin is used to treat *Mycobacterium tuberculosis*. Neomycin is used for topical wound irrigation.

The worst side effect associated with aminoglycosides is damage to renal tubules. Dizziness and nausea may also occur.

Tetracyclines

Tetracyclines can be bacteriostatic or bacterici-dal, depending on the dose—like a chameleon! Tetracyclines act by screwing up bacterial wall synthesis. You can tell when the antibiotic is a tetracycline, because the name ends in cycline! Too clever.

They're effective in treating *Mycoplasma* infection and atypical pneumonias.

Side effects include gastrointestinal irritation with nausea, vomiting, and diarrhea, bone mar-row depression, and hypersensitivity reactions.

*Q*9. Tetracyclines are incorporated into the liver and kidney for a while, so be careful using them in patients with _____ or _____ disease.

Use of these drugs in kids with developing teeth causes tooth discoloration. They also permanently affect skeletal bones, retarding growth.

Q10. List three patient populations in which tetracyclines should be used cautiously, if at all.
1. _____
2. _____
3. _____

Fluoroquinolones

Fluoroquinolones are broad spectrum with increased potency against gram-negative organisms. They act by inhibiting bacterial DNA synthesis. This group of drugs is especially useful in treating infections associated with chronic bronchitic and cystic fibrosis.

Polymyxins

Polymyxin B and E are the two drugs in the polymyxin category. Polymyxins are good for fighting gram-negative organisms and *Pseudomonas* organisms, but they're really toxic to the kidneys and nerves. As a result, their use is limited to topical ointment.

Macrolide Antibiotics (Erythromycins)

Macrolide antibiotics inhibit protein synthesis, so the microorganism is thwarted! Macrolides are used for respiratory, gastrointestinal, genital, and skin/soft tissue infections. They are the drug of choice for treating *Mycoplasma* and *Legionella* organisms. It's nice to be tops in your chosen field!

Now, to see if you've been paying attention (not that I would doubt you), I'll give you a disease or an infection, and you give me an appropriate antibiotic to treat it. Sounds like fun, doesn't it!?

Q11. *Pseudomonas aeruginosa*
_____

Q12. *Mycobacterium tuberculosis*
_____

Q13. *Mycoplasma pneumoniae*
_____

Q14. *Klebsiella* infection
_____

Q15. Gram-positive cocci
_____

Q16. *Legionella* pneumonia
_____

Antifungal Agents

Yuk! Whose idea was it to include this stuff? Did you know that you have fungus in the back of your throat (*Candida albicans*), in your sputum and stools, etc.? The point is, the presence of fungi is no big deal. The problem arises if you're immunocompromised or taking broad-spectrum antibiotics. (Antibiotics screw up the balance of normal flora.) Let's look at a couple of the most common antifungal drugs.

List two or three patient populations who are immunocompromised.
_____
_____

Answer: Patients with AIDS, organ transplant recipients, and patients receiving chemotherapy are a few examples.

Remember how we talked (in a previous chapter) about how corticosteroids given via MDI could cause oral candidiasis? Well, that happens because the drug upsets the balance of normal flora by being deposited in the oropharynx.

Q17. How do you minimize this?
_____
_____

Amphotericin B

Since amphotericin B is relatively toxic (nephrotoxicity, fever, hypotension), it's not used a lot. It increases the permeability of the fungal cell membrane, which allows ions and small molecules to leak out of the cell.

Azole Antifungal Agents

Azole antifungal agents are an alternative to amphotericin B in treating fungal infections. Azole agents increase cell membrane permeability, essential cell components leak out, and the cell dies.

It's like if your body's permeability got altered and your liver leaked out . . . sort of.

The following are adverse effects of azole antifungal agents:

- Nausea/vomiting/diarrhea
- Abdominal pain
- Abnormal liver function
- Headache
- Fatigue
- Rash

Antituberculosis Agents

Multiple-drug therapy is used to treat TB. "First-line" drug therapy for 9 months:

- Isoniazid and rifampin for 9 months
- Ethambutol, streptomycin, or pyrazinamide for the initial 2- to 8-week treatment period

Using either of the above combinations, a relapse rate of 0% to 4% has been noted. (Management of TB is considered effective in the United States and Canada if the relapse rate is less than 5%.)

The following combo has also been tried:

- Isoniazid, rifampin, pyrazinamide, and either ethambutol or streptomycin for 2 months, followed by isoniazid and rifampin for 4 months

Think of several settings or situations where TB might occur (low socioeconomic status, immunocompromised, etc.).

*Q*18. How do you think compliance might be affected with the above regimens?

_____

_____

_____

_____

Drug-resistant Tuberculosis

It's not really clear how prevalent multiple-drug resistant TB is. If a patient exhibits resistance to one of the drugs in the regimen, another is substituted. The cure rate for multiple-drug resistant TB is poor.

Antiviral Agents

There are some nasty viruses out there (AIDS, influenza, RSV), so it would be nice if we had a pill or something!

Protease Inhibitors

You've probably heard of protease inhibitors as the latest in HIV treatment. They act by inhibiting enzyme activity necessary to make mature infectious particles. They're helpful, but not curative.

Indicate whether the following statements are true or false.

_____ *Q*19. HIV can be cured by protease inhibitors.

*Q*20. Resistance to a drug in the TB regimen has a poor prognosis.

_____

What! You want even more questions!? Okay, but remember, you begged me.

1. Which of the following is a substance produced by microorganisms, capable of inhibiting or killing bacteria and other microorganisms?
   a. Antiinfective
   b. Antimicrobial
   c. Antibiotic
   d. Bacteriolytic   (Chapter 14, p. 247)

2. Antibiotics can act by which of the following mechanisms?
   I.   Inhibition of cell wall synthesis
   II. Alteration of cell membrane permeability
   III. Inhibition of protein synthesis
   IV. Inhibition of DNA synthesis

   a. I, II, III, IV
   b. I, II, III
   c. II, III, IV
   d. I, III, IV   (Chapter 14, p. 248)

3. Which of the following describes antibiotics that are useful against a wide range of organisms?
   a. Narrow-spectrum
   b. Broad-spectrum
   c. Efficacious
   d. Resistant   (Chapter 14, p. 249)

4. Which of the following is an enzyme produced by bacteria that can inactivate an antibiotic?
   a. Monobactase
   b. Carbapenase
   c. Penicillinase
   d. Alpha-lactamase (Chapter 14, p. 250)

5. All but which of the following are beta-lactam antibiotics?
   a. Penicillin
   b. Cephalosporin
   c. Carbapenem
   d. Aminoglycoside (Chapter 14, p. 250)

6. Which of the following antibiotics should be used cautiously in children because of the effect on skeletal growth?
   a. Beta-lactams
   b. Aminoglycosides
   c. Tetracyclines
   d. Quinolones   (Chapter 14, p. 254)

7. All but which of the following is true of polymyxin antibiotics?
   a. They are effective in treating *Pseudomonas* infection.
   b. They are effective in fighting gram-positive bacteria.
   c. They are toxic to kidneys and nerves.
   d. They are used as a topical ointment.
                        (Chapter 14, p. 255)

8. Which of the following is a fungal disease that may occur in the oropharynx when steroids are administered via MDI?
   a. Oral candidiasis
   b. *Chlamydia* infection
   c. *Aspergillus* infection
   d. Blastomycosis   (Chapter 14, p. 257)

9. Which antifungal drug is the least toxic alternative to treat invasive fungal disease?
   a. Amphotericin B
   b. Nystatin
   c. Flucytosine
   d. Azole agents   (Chapter 14, p. 258)

10. All but which of the following is true of the treatment of TB?
   a. Resistance to one of the drugs in the regimen leads to a poor prognosis.
   b. Multiple drugs are used.
   c. Drug therapy is prescribed for 6 or 9 months.
   d. Resistance to multiple drugs in the regimen leads to a poor prognosis.
                        (Chapter 14, pp. 258-260)

Sim

Mr. Green has been diagnosed with TB. He lives in a homeless shelter on 133rd and Lexington. What treatment regimen would you recommend for him?

_____

_____

_____

_____

Answer: Because compliance may be an issue for Mr. Green, I'd go for the 6-month regimen instead of the 9-month regimen. Let's say isoniazid, rifampin, pyrazinamide, and ethambutol for 2 months, followed by isoniazid and rifampin for 4 months.

Resistance to ethambutol is not uncommon, and Mr. Green is indeed resistant to this drug. What do you do now?

_____

_____

Answer: Replace it with streptomycin.

How are you going to get across to Mr. Green the importance of taking his meds for 6 months?

_____

_____

_____

_____

Answer: This is one of those unanswerable questions but worth thinking about. He may comply, and then again, he may not. In the scheme of things, this just may not be that important to him. Something to remember, though, is that you probably have no idea what it's like to be Mr. Green, so tread carefully. He may be able to show up at a clinic, pick up his meds, and get a free sandwich or something to that effect. What motivates Mr. Green?

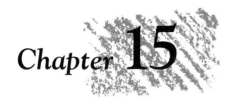

Chapter 15 Cold and Cough Agents

What's a cold, anyway? I'm glad you asked that question. It's defined as a nonbacterial upper respiratory infection characterized by mild general malaise (not captain malaise) and a runny, stuffy nose. Other symptoms might include sneezing, sore throat, cough, and some chest discomfort.

On the other hand, the flu is associated with a fever, headache, muscle ache, and extreme fatigue and weakness. Onset of symptoms is usually rapid.

Drug Classes

There are four classes of drugs in cold remedies, used by themselves or in combination.

Sympathomimetic (Adrenergic) Decongestants
Do sympathomimetic (adrenergic) decongestants sound familiar? If not, close your book and use it for a door stop. In the case of colds, sympathomimetics are used for their vasoconstriction effect (alpha stimulation), resulting in decongestion. They can be taken orally or used as topical sprays (Neo-Synephrine, Sinex).

Onset is quicker with topical application (sniffing it), but if you do this repeatedly, you'll get swollen mucosa. So only use it for a few days at a time. Afrin can actually cause tolerance and withdrawal symptoms when you quit!

   $\mathcal{Q}$1. If you take the drug orally, you may get some beta-1 effects, which are _____ and _____ .

Antihistamines
Recall that histamine is one of the mediators of local inflammatory responses? Specifically, H_1 receptors, involved in inflammation and allergic reactions, produce skin reactions, bronchoconstriction, mucus secretion, nasal congestion, and irritation.

   $\mathcal{Q}$2. The typical antihistamine found in cold remedies is an H_1 receptor agonist. It blocks the bronchopulmonary and vascular actions of histamine, preventing

   _____

   _____

A partial list of examples of H_1 receptor agonists follows:

- Benadryl
- Chlor-Trimeton
- Hismanal
- Tavist
- Seldane
- Claritin

Antihistamines have three effects:
1. Antihistaminic—block bronchial smooth muscle constriction caused by histamine
2. Sedative—antihistamines cross into the brain
3. Anticholinergic—upper airway drying

Certain CNS effects like anxiety, stimulation, and nervousness may also occur. These effects are less likely to occur with occasional use (like with a cold).

Depending on the antihistamine, the duration lasts anywhere from 4 to 6 to 12 hours (nonsedating brands). The nonsedating brands don't have the anticholinergic effects either.

Q 3. One of the great effects of antihistamines if you have a cold is that drying effect, so your nose doesn't run all day. But what could be a drawback to this? _____

_____

Answer: Secretions are an airway defense mechanism. Antihistamines might impair secretion clearance and lead to impacted secretions. Eeew! Be certain that your patient has adequate hydration!

Second-generation H_1 receptor antagonists that are more useful than first generation antihistamines in the treatment of seasonal allergic rhinitis. They're better tolerated, have fewer side effects, and last longer.

Expectorants

Expectorants facilitate removal of secretions from the lower respiratory tract. There are two types (as if you care):

Mucolytic expectorants—drugs that facilitate removal of mucus by mucolytic action (like acetylcysteine [Mucomyst])

Stimulant expectorants—drugs that increase the production (and presumably clearance) of mucus in the respiratory tract (guaifenesin [Robitussin], etc.)

Generally, stimulant expectorants are what is meant when we talk about cold medicine.

Hey, I bet you never thought of this. If a cold involves the upper respiratory tract, why are expectorants used to treat them? Think about it.

_____

_____

_____

Answer: Since mucus incorporates water as it's produced, adequate intake of plain water, milk, fruit juice, etc., helps preserve the viscosity and clearance of mucus. So if you have a simple cold, drink up!

Cough Suppressants (Antitussives)

Remember, coughing is a defense mechanism, so why (under what circumstances) would you want to thwart it? _____

Answer: You want to still a dry, hacking, non-productive coughing or coughing that interferes with sleep.

Vagal stimulation in the larynx and bronchi and even the stomach (who knew?) can cause a cough. This also increases bronchial secretions.

Cough suppressants act by suppressing the cough center in the medulla; narcotics do an awfully nice job of this. Common examples are codeine (narcotic) and dextromethorphan (nonnarcotic). These are the two most common cough suppressants, based on both safety and efficacy. Many cough suppressants contain codeine.

In the adult:

- 10 to 20 mg—cough suppression
- More than 30 mg—analgesic effect

You can get both codeine and dextromethorphan OTC.

If your patient has lots of copious secretions (cystic fibrosis, chronic bronchitis), it's a bad idea to suppress the patient's cough.

Here's another thing that has always bothered me. What about preparations that contain both an expectorant and a cough suppressant? It's like Rhode Island. It's neither a road nor an island. Discuss.

Answer: The rationale for the above combo (not Rhode Island) is that it's better to have a less frequent, productive cough than a frequent, dry cough. Anyway.

Cold Compounds

Many cold remedies contain alcohol as the solvent. Nyquil Nighttime Cold/Flu Medicine is 25% alcohol! Contac Severe Cold/Flu Nighttime Liquid has 18.5% alcohol!

In many instances, OTC remedies have the same ingredients as the prescription formula, only in lower concentrations.

Treating a Cold

Starve a cold, feed a fever. No, feed a cold, starve a fever. No, *you can't cure a cold, so treat the symptoms and forget about the food!*

Every ingredient in cold remedies has potential problems, so remember to consider the potential problems posed by each ingredient. And by the way, write them in the following blanks.

Q 4. Sympathomimetics _____

Q 5. Antihistamines _____

Q 6. Expectorants _____

Q 7. Antitussives _____

Don't forget fluids, rest, chicken soup, and NBRC questions.

1. The common cold is described by all but which of the following?
   a. Lower respiratory tract infection
   b. Upper respiratory infection
   c. Nonbacterial
   d. Characterized by mild malaise
   (Chapter 15, p. 265)

2. Regarding sympathomimetic decongestants, which method of administration gives the fastest relief?
   a. Oral
   b. Topical
   c. IM
   d. a and b are equal (Chapter 15, p. 265)

3. Systemic side effects associated with sympathomimetic decongestants include which of the following?
   I. Increased minute volume
   II. Increased blood pressure
   III. Increased heart rate
   IV. Increased sputum production

   a. I, II, III
   b. II and III
   c. II, III, IV
   d. I and IV   (Chapter 15, p. 266)

4. H_1 histamine receptors accomplish which of the following?
   a. Block allergic reactions
   b. Desensitize inflammatory cells
   c. Stabilize mast cells
   d. Cause inflammation
   (Chapter 15, p. 267)

5. Which of the following is the typical antihistamine found in cold medications?
   a. H_1 receptor agonist
   b. H_1 receptor antagonist
   c. H_2 receptor agonist
   d. H_2 receptor antagonist
   (Chapter 15, p. 267)

6. Which of the following are effects of antihistamines?
   a. Sedative
   b. Antihistaminic
   c. Anticholinergic
   d. All the above   (Chapter 15, p. 268)

7. What is the duration of action for nonsedating antihistamines?
   a. 2 to 4 hours
   b. 4 to 6 hours
   c. 8 to 10 hours
   d. 12 hours   (Chapter 15, p. 268)

8. Expectorants facilitate removal of mucus from which of the following?
   a. Upper respiratory tract
   b. Sinuses
   c. Lower respiratory tract
   d. a and b   (Chapter 15, p. 270)

9. Cough suppressants accomplish which of the following?
   a. Act on the cerebral cortex
   b. Stimulate vagal receptors
   c. Depress the medulla's cough center
   d. Block vagal sensory endings
                              (Chapter 15, p. 271)

10. The cough reflex should *not* be suppressed in which of the following?
    a. Patients with cystic fibrosis
    b. Patients with chronic bronchitis
    c. Patients with pneumonia
    d. a and b   (Chapter 15, p. 272)

Sim
You are baby-sitting your little brother, who has a runny nose, is sneezing, and says he feels "icky." You take his temperature (98.8° F). What's your differential diagnosis?

_____

Answer: He has the classic symptoms of a cold.

What treatment would help him the most at present?

_____
_____

Answer: Just like Mom always said, rest, plenty of fluids, and maybe a nasal decongestant for the runny nose.

He later develops a cough that is dry and nonproductive; his temperature is still normal. Anything you would/should change with your treatment regimen? _____
_____
_____

Answer: If the temperature is normal, he's not lethargic, and he doesn't complain of a headache, he's still got a cold. Since the cough is dry and nonproductive, there's no use making him hack in vain, so add a cough suppressant (antitussive if you want to impress the pharmacist) to your list. The antitussive will also be good so the little dear can rest without being awakened by coughing. This way he can get his strength back to hassle you in a few short days!

Chapter 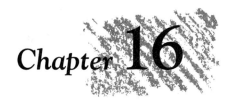 16 Selected Agents Used in Respiratory Disease

In this chapter we'll look at three groups of drugs used for the direct treatment or prevention of respiratory disease.

Alpha-1-Proteinase Inhibitor (Human)

Alpha-1-proteinase inhibitor is abbreviated as API, so don't think I'll ever write it out again! It's also known as alpha-1 antitrypsin. It's used to treat congenital alpha-1 antitrypsin deficiency, which ultimately leads to emphysema.

The product is called prolastin. It's made from pooled human plasma from healthy donors, and goes through all the usual purification and treatment to get the infectious gunk out of it.

Alpha-1 Antitrypsin Deficiency

Alpha-1 antitrypsin deficiency is a genetic defect that can lead to panacinar emphysema, usually between the ages of 30 and 50. It accounts for about 2% of all emphysema in the United States. It's worse in the lower lung zones and can be accelerated by cigarette smoking—yet another reason to stay away from cigarettes.

Normally, there's an enzyme called neutrophil elastase that can burn through alveolar walls. Elastase is held in check by alpha-1 antitrypsin. If there's a *deficiency* in alpha-1 antitrypsin, the elastase goes on a rampage, alveolar walls are destroyed, and the result is emphysema.

Prolastin therapy is indicated as long-term replacement therapy in patients who have a congenital alpha-1 antitrypsin deficiency, with clinically demonstrated panacinar emphysema.

By the time you get panacinar emphysema, your lungs have sustained structural damage, and prolastin won't reverse the damage, or improve lung function. Once your alveolar walls are gone, there's nothing you can do about it.

Q1. Explain the sequence of events leading to panacinar emphysema caused by alpha-1 antitrypsin deficiency. _____
_____
_____
_____

Guess how much prolastin costs. _____

Answer: $25,000 to $40,000 per year. It ain't cheap!

Dose and Administration

Because so few patients have alpha-1 antitrypsin deficiency, prolastin is considered an orphan drug. The recommended dose is 60 mg/kg body weight, once a week. It's given IV at a rate of 0.8 ml/kg/min or greater. The total infusion takes about 30 minutes.

Q2. Calculate a dose using your own weight.
_____

Hazards and Side Effects

Prolastin is basically well tolerated, but the following side effects do occur:

- Fever
- Light-headedness
- Dyspnea
- Tachycardia (rare)
- Dizziness
- Flulike symptoms
- Rash
- Hypotension (rare)

Nicotine Replacement Therapy

The response to nicotine is both sympathetic and parasympathetic:

Sympathetic

- Hypertension, tachycardia, peripheral vaso-constriction (remember "fight or flight"?)
- Release of epinephrine

Parasympathetic

- Nausea, vomiting, diarrhea, urination

Response to nicotine is dose dependent. Nicotine also binds to receptors in the CNS, causing the following:

- Respiratory stimulation
- Tremors
- Convulsions
- Nausea and emesis

The CNS stimulation is what appears to provide nicotine's positive reinforcement in smokers. There is increased alertness and cognitive performance (at lower doses) and a positive euphoric effect (at higher doses).

Q3. Have you or someone you know quit (or tried to quit) smoking? _____

Q4. What symptoms did you or that someone experience? How did you or that someone feel?

_____
_____
_____

Withdrawal from nicotine is a bear (as you can attest to if you or someone you know well has gone through it). The smoker loses the stimulatory and euphoric effects, not to mention physical withdrawal symptoms. In its ability to addict, nicotine is similar to heroin. Many people think that all it takes to quit is will power, but for lots of people, will power isn't enough.

Withdrawal symptoms include the following:

- Craving for nicotine
- Anxiety
- Impaired concentration
- Nervousness, irritability
- Sleep disturbances or drowsiness
- Increased appetite/ weight gain

Be aware of these symptoms in your hospitalized patients. Many of them are going through nicotine withdrawal, and their symptoms are attributed to something else altogether.

Nicotine replacement therapy is intended to assist the smoker with smoking cessation by allowing gradual withdrawal from nicotine. This therapy is available in a transdermal patch, a polacrilex gum, and a nasal spray.

Indications
- An aid to smoking cessation to relieve the symptoms of nicotine withdrawal

Replacement therapy should be used along with behavioral modification to increase compliance and minimize the chances of relapse.

How can you tell if the patient has a strong addiction to nicotine?

- Smoking more than 15 cigarettes a day
- Preference for brands with nicotine levels higher than 0.9 mg
- Inhaling smoke frequently and deeply
- Smoking within 30 minutes of getting up in the morning
- Can't give up that first morning cigarette and smokes more frequently in the AM

Q5. Construct a profile of the world's most addicted smoker—no names, please!

_____
_____
_____
_____

Formulations

Nicotine polacrilex gum

Nicotine polacrilex gum contains nicotine resin in a chewing gum base. It's hard to chew, may cause aching jaws, and tastes bad. (That's not exactly a ringing endorsement for smoking cessation!) Absorption of the nicotine is faster with gum than with the patch, which is an advantage for some smokers.

The nicotine isn't absorbed as well if you drink acidic beverages (coffee, soda, orange juice) while you're chewing it. Here's how it works:

1. Chew the gum until it's malleable.

2. "Park" it between the cheek and gum.

3. Wait until the taste is gone.

4. Repeat the entire sequence.

Intermittent chewing like this slows absorption of the nicotine that's being released, so less nicotine is swallowed. If you swallow too much nicotine, you'll be sick (surprise).

Dose

Nicotine gum comes as 2-mg (recommended for those who smoke less than 25 cigarettes a day) and 4-mg strength (for those who smoke more than 25 cigarettes a day). The first 6 weeks, chew a piece every 1 to 2 hours; weeks 7 through 9, every 2 to 4 hours; weeks 10 through 12, every 4 to 8 hours.

Nicotine Transdermal System

A nicotine transdermal system consists of a multilayered patch that delivers nicotine for 24 hours after it's applied to the skin. Somewhere around 68% of the nicotine that is released actually enters the circulation.

With Nicoderm, blood levels of nicotine rise quickly and then plateau for 2 to 4 hours; with Habitrol, blood levels peak between 6 and 12 hours and then decline. Patches come in various strengths depending on the brand. Stronger

doses of nicotine (21 mg) are given initially, and then the dose is tapered (maybe to 7 mg). The 21-mg strength is about the same as half a pack per day.

Precautions

Precautions include not using more than one patch and not smoking while the patch is being worn. Some patients feel like they need more nicotine, so they wear more patches, or smoke while they have a patch on. Too much nicotine may cause nausea, vomiting, and cardiac dysrhythmias. And don't ever light one. (That was a joke, don't highlight it.)

A common side effect is skin irritation at the site of the patch. Rotating the site takes care of this.

Nicotine Nasal Spray

Nasal spray produces rapid peak plasma levels of nicotine because it delivers the drug directly to the nasal membranes. Irritant effects include runny nose, nasal irritation, sneezing, cough, and watery eyes. It comes as 0.5 mg per spray—one per nostril. Patients may take up to 5 doses per hour or 40 doses per day (seems like a lot), reducing the dose over 4 to 6 weeks.

*Q*6. List one advantage and one disadvantage of each nicotine replacement formulation.

	Advantage	Disadvantage
Nicotine gum		
Nicotine patch		
Nicotine nasal spray		

Precautions

- Don't use nicotine replacement products longer than 3 months. It's possible to transfer addiction from cigarettes to the smoking cessation product.
- Be careful about using it in patients with cardiovascular disease, coronary artery disease, dysrhythmias, or hypertension.

Q7. In addition, if a patient is wearing the patch, what should the patient be cautioned *not* to do? _____

_____

Q8. What can happen if the patient wears too many patches? _____

_____

Nitric Oxide

Nitric oxide is a vasodilator that is being studied because of its ability to lower PVR in persistent pulmonary hypertension of the newborn and ARDS. It's an orphan drug.

Nitric oxide diffuses easily into the blood stream, is inactivated by binding to hemoglobin, acts on the pulmonary vascular endothelium (and *only* here), and causes selective pulmonary vasodilation.

Q9. If my patient inhaled exogenous nitric oxide, could vasodilation occur systemically? _____

Toxicity
Toxicity can be caused by the following:

• The nitric oxide itself
• Formation of the nitrate, NO_2
• Formation of methemoglobin

The amount of NO_2 produced depends on the amount of nitric oxide and the surrounding oxygen. The higher the FiO_2, the greater the amount of oxidation from nitric oxide to NO_2.

The lethal effect of NO_2 is due to pulmonary edema. In usual doses (0.5% to 4%), methemoglobinemia is generally not a problem.

Q10. What's a good thing about nitric oxide?

_____

_____

Q11. What's a bad thing? _____

_____

Administration
Nitric oxide is administered as a gas in concentrations up to 80 parts per million (ppm). Most doses are less than or equal to 10 ppm. Nitric oxide is delivered to ventilated lung units and doesn't increase ventilation-perfusion mismatch (which would cause worsening of hypoxemia).

Because nitric oxide is locally and quickly inactivated by hemoglobin, there's no systemic vasodilation or hypotension.

When you try to wean a patient from nitric oxide, do it gradually to prevent pulmonary hypertension and/or arterial desaturation. The vasodilating effect of nitric oxide ends when you remove the gas. You may need to give the patient more oxygen as nitric oxide is withdrawn. Given this, what parameters should be monitored when administering nitric oxide therapy?

_____

_____

Answer: PaO_2 or SpO_2, pulmonary artery pressures (patient must have a Swan-Ganz catheter), vital signs (VS).

Ready to forge ahead with the NBRCs? Let's do it anyway.

1. Prolastin is prepared by which of the following?
   a. Synthetically
   b. Naturally
   c. Using both natural and synthetic products
   d. In a vacuum.   (Chapter 16, p. 276)

2. All but which of the following statements are true about prolastin?
   a. It is an orphan drug.
   b. It is expensive.
   c. It is used to treat alpha-1 antitrypsin deficiency.
   d. It reverses damage done by panacinar emphysema.   (Chapter 16, p. 276)

3. Which of the following are true of Alpha-1 antitrypsin deficiency?
   I.   It's genetic.
   II. It causes centrilobular emphysema.
   III. It accounts for the majority of emphysema cases in the United States.
   IV. It presents as emphysema between the ages of 30 and 50.

   a. I, II, III, IV
   b. I, II, III
   c. I, IV
   d. II, III   (Chapter 16, pp. 275-276)

4. The enzyme responsible for destroying connective tissue in the alveoli and for causing emphysema is which of the following?
   a. Cholinesterase
   b. Elastase
   c. Emphysemase
   d. Antiprotease   (Chapter 16, p. 276)

5. Nicotine affects which of the following?
   a. SNS
   b. PSN
   c. CNS
   d. All the above   (Chapter 16, p. 277)

6. Nicotine replacement therapy is available in all but which of the following formulations?
   a. Tablets
   b. Gum
   c. Transdermal patch
   d. Nasal spray   (Chapter 16, p. 278)

7. Which of the following indicates a strong physical dependence on nicotine?
   a. Not inhaling
   b. Smoking 5 to 10 cigarettes per day
   c. Difficulty in giving up the first morning cigarette
   d. Smoking low nicotine brands
                       (Chapter 16, p. 278)

8. Which of the following describes nicotine polacrilex gum?
   a. Has a pleasant taste
   b. Is easy to chew
   c. Is better absorbed if taken with orange juice
   d. Is available in two strengths
                       (Chapter 16, p. 279)

9. Nicotine replacement therapy should be gradually withdrawn and stopped by which of the following?
   a. 1 month
   b. 2 months
   c. 3 months
   d. 4 months   (Chapter 16, p. 279)

10. Which of the following describes nitric oxide?
    a. Is a systemic vasodilator
    b. Lowers pulmonary vascular resistance
    c. Is used to treat high blood pressure
    d. Is associated with refractory hypoxemia   (Chapter 16, p. 279)

Sim

You are conducting a smoking cessation class at a local lung association. One of the participants is the president of a local university. She puts in an average of 60 hr/week and is highly visible. She uses smoking as a means to reduce stress but wants to quit. She asks you to recommend the method that would best suit her lifestyle.

_____

_____

_____

_____

Answer: Stress to her that she remain in your classes. Smoking cessation is accomplished on many levels, using behavior modification, group counseling, and education. Because she is such a public presence, chewing gum or inhaling a spray several times a day would be too conspicuous! Recommend the transdermal patch (as long as she has no history of cardiovascular disease).

Your patient is a heavy smoker (about 40 cigarettes a day). Any other advice and/or instructions for her?

_____
_____
_____
_____

Answer: Yes. (Or else I wouldn't have asked the question!). Begin with the highest dose (21 mg) and gradually taper to 7 mg/day. This should be accomplished in no more than 3 months. Caution her not to smoke while she is wearing the patch. Educate her as to what withdrawal symptoms she can expect. Let her know that they will pass and teach her some coping techniques. Make sure she alternates the site of her patches so that she isn't bothered by skin irritation.

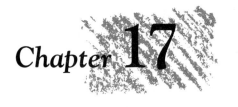

Chapter 17 Aerosolized Drug Delivery in Neonates and Children

Guess what we're going to discuss in this chapter?!

Factors Affecting Drug Therapy in Neonates and Children

When administering drug therapy, remember that babies and children aren't just small adults. Although size is certainly one difference between children and adults that also affects drug therapy, other factors include a lack of receptors for certain drugs or a lack of enzymes to break down a drug (producing toxic effects). Here's what you should be called, based on your age:

- Premature neonate—younger than 36 weeks' gestation
- Neonate—first 4 weeks of postnatal life
- Infant—1 to 12 months
- Child—1 to 12 years
- Adolescent—12 to 18 years
- Adult—older than 18 years

Pharmaceutical Factors
Dosage form and route of administration must take age into account. Infants can't swallow a pill, etc.

*Q*1. List two instances where age and route of administration are incompatible.
  1. _____
  2. _____

*Q*2. List one or two routes of administration that are applicable to any age.
  1. _____
  2. _____

Pharmacokinetic Factors
Neonates and children differ from adults in the absorption, distribution, metabolism, and elimination of drugs. The following lists total body water as a percentage of weight:

- 85% in the premature neonate
- 70% in the full-term infant
- 65% in the child
- 60% in the adult

The following lists extracellular fluid as a percentage of weight:

- 50% in the premature neonate
- 40% in the full-term infant
- 25% in the child
- 15% in the adult

*Q*3. Circle one. Total body water and extracellular fluid affect the distribution of (water-soluble, lipid-soluble) drugs.

Glomerular filtration rate and tubular function are immature in the neonate and take about 6 months to fully develop.

*Q*4. Decreased renal clearance _____ the ability of neonates to get rid of drug metabolites in urine, requiring dosage adjustments of lots of drugs.

Pharmacodynamic Factors

Infants and children often respond differently than adults to certain drugs, as well as movie and book selections. For example, methylphenidate (Ritalin) (a CNS stimulant in the adult) actually increases attention span and decreases disruptive behavior in hyperactive children.

Calculating Pediatric Doses

Always check the product literature, *PDR*, *Pediatric Dosage Handbook*, *Manual of Pediatric Therapeutics*, or the *Harriet Lane Handbook* to see if there's already a recommended, established pediatric dose. If there isn't one, there's a way to estimate the correct dose (lucky you). In fact, you have your choice of four! Just like Christmas, isn't it (or Hannukah, or Kwanza, or your birthday)?

1. Fried's rule (for infants younger than 1 year)

$$\text{Infant dose} = \frac{\text{Infant age (months)}}{150 \text{ months}} \times \text{Adult dose}$$

2. Young's rule (1 to 12 years)

$$\text{Child dose} = \frac{\text{Child's age (years)}}{\text{child's age} + 12} \times \text{Adult dose}$$

3. Clark's rule

$$\text{Child dose} = \frac{\text{Child's weight (pounds)}}{150 \text{ pounds}} \times \text{Adult dose}$$

4. Body Surface Area (BSA)

$$\text{Child dose} = \frac{\text{Child BSA (m}^2)}{1.73} \times \text{Adult dose}$$

You can get BSA from a nomogram using the child's weight and height. Even though you may not have one lying around the house, your pediatrician has one.

$\mathcal{Q}$5. Calculate the dose of loratadine (Claritin) for a 10-year-old. Adult dose is 10 mg.

_____

Because so many variables can affect drug action in neonates and children, watch the pediatric patient closely, especially the first time you give the dose.

Pediatric Doses of Aerosolized Drugs

Some bronchoactive drugs are not approved for use in children younger than 12 years, but most of them are approved by the FDA for use in kids. Sympathomimetics approved for use in pediatric patients include the following:

- Racemic epinephrine
- Isoetharine
- Terbutaline
- Bitolterol
- Salmeterol
- Isoproterenol
- Metaproterenol
- Albuterol
- Pirbuterol

Approved anticholinergic bronchodilators:
- Atropine
- Ipratropium

Mucolytics:
- Acetylcysteine
- Dornase alfa

Corticosteroids:
- Dexamethasone
- Flunisolide
- Beclomethasone
- Fluticasone

Antiasthmatics:
- Cromolyn sodium
- Nedocromil sodium

Antiinfectives:
- Ribavirin
- Pentamidine

Because the doses are smaller for pediatric patients, you may have to add more diluent to get enough volume for the SVN. Does this dilute the dose? (Check Chapter 4 if you don't remember.) ————————————

_____

Answer: The drug is not diluted, because the same amount is delivered. It is, however, expanded.

For aerosolized bronchodilators, the adult dose is often prescribed for a neonate. This may be because of the immature development of smooth muscle and receptors, which is normal for infants and would require a higher dose to get the desired effect.

Pediatric Aerosol Administration

Aerosols are the logical route of administration for treating the lungs and airways of pediatric patients. The following table gives you some general guidelines on age requirements for using various delivery devices to give aerosolized drugs.

Delivery Method	Minimum Age
SVN	neonate
MDI	>5 yr
With spacer	>4 yr
With spacer and mask	infant
With endotracheal tube	neonate
Breath-actuated MDI	>5 yr
DPI	≥5 yr

Based on the National Asthma Education and Prevention Program Guidelines, 1997.

DPI, Dry powder inhaler; *MDI*, metered dose inhaler; *SVN*, small volume nebulizer.

Q 6. As with adults, about ———— % of the aerosolized drug reaches the lungs.

Do you remember why the DPI probably can't be used in kids younger than 5 years?

_____

_____

Answer: The patient must be able to generate a minimal flow rate of 60 L/min, which is difficult or impossible for little kids.

SVNs are usually given with a face mask that the caregiver, parent, or child can hold, pretending to be a space man (space person is more politically correct), pilot, etc. Use your imagination for this—but not to answer the NBRC questions!

1. A person in the first 4 weeks of postnatal life is correctly termed which of the following?
   a. Postmature neonate
   b. Neonate
   c. Infant
   d. Baby   (Chapter 17, p. 284)

2. Which of the following describes when total body water as a percentage of weight decreases?
   a. As age increases
   b. As age decreases
   c. As renal function improves
   d. As glomerular filtration deteriorates
                    (Chapter 17, p. 284)

3. In the neonate/infant, which of the following describes when renal function is fully developed?
   a. 1 month
   b. 3 months
   c. 6 months
   d. 1 year   (Chapter 17, p. 284)

4. Which of the following can be used to calculate pediatric drug dosages?
   I.   Drug product information
   II. Young's rule
   III. Fried's rule
   IV. Canne's rule

   a. I, II, III, IV
   b. I, II, III
   c. II, III, IV
   d. I, III, IV   (Chapter 17, p. 284)

5. Which of the following is the route of administration of choice for delivering medication to the lungs of a child?
   a. IV
   b. Topical
   c. Oral
   d. Aerosol   (Chapter 17, p. 285)

6. Which aerosol delivery devices can be used to treat a neonate?
   a. SVN
   b. MDI through endotracheal tube
   c. MDI with spacer
   d. a and b   (Chapter 17, p. 287)

7. Which aerosol delivery devices can be used to treat a 5-year-old patient?
   a. SVN
   b. MDI with spacer
   c. DPI
   d. All the above   (Chapter 17, p. 287)

8. Which of the following applies to a DPI?
   a. Require that the user generate 60 to 120 L/min of flow
   b. Should only be used with a spacer
   c. Can be done through the endotracheal tube
   d. All the above
      (Chapter 17, pp. 285-287)

9. Factors that affect drug therapy include which of the following?
   a. Size and weight
   b. Mass and volume
   c. Temperature and pressure
   d. Size and age   (Chapter 17, p. 283)

10. A route of administration that works well at any age includes which of the following?
    a. Oral
    b. Topical
    c. IV
    d. Injection   (Chapter 17, p. 287)

Sim

An 18-month-old child is to receive metaproterenol via aerosol therapy. What delivery devices are available to you?

_____
_____
_____

Answer: SVN, MDI with spacer and mask, MDI with endotracheal tube.

The child is not intubated. Which method would you select? Justify your selection.

_____
_____
_____

Answer: You could choose either SVN or MDI with spacer and mask as long as you provide good reasons. I would choose SVN, based only on the child's age. Most 18-month-old kids will tolerate a mask held loosely against their face as long as you're making a game of it. The same rule also applies in peds. With SVN you've got many more chances (breaths) to deliver the meds; with MDI, you've only got two or three shots.

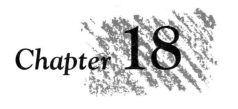

Chapter 18 Skeletal Muscle Relaxants (Neuromuscular Blocking Agents)

Neuromuscular blocking agents (muscle relaxants) have the ability to cause skeletal muscle paralysis if they're given in high enough doses. There are two types: depolarizing and nondepolarizing.

South American Indians used to use curare as arrow poison. We still use this today as a nondepolarizing paralyzing agent. Who knew you'd get a history tidbit for free!

Use

Neuromuscular blocking agents are used clinically for the following reasons:
• To facilitate endotracheal intubation
• For muscle paralysis during surgery
• To facilitate mechanical ventilation (like if the patient is "fighting" the ventilator)

They're usually given IV, although it's quite a visual to imagine the doctors shooting patients with curare-tipped arrows!

Q1. The effects are dose related, so if you give a small dose, you get a _____ effect.

In the operating suite neuromuscular blocking agents are used as part of the anesthesia before they intubate you.

In the ICU the agents are used for elective intubation or in the management of certain patients receiving ventilation.

Physiology of Neuromuscular Junction

One of the branches of the peripheral nervous system—the somatic, or skeletal, muscle—contains striated muscle.

Q2. Give two or three examples of skeletal muscle.

_____

_____

Did you list the diaphragm?

The interface of nerve fiber and skeletal muscle is called the neuromuscular or myoneural junction. Remember, acetylcholine is the neurotransmitter at the neuromuscular junction.

In the *depolarization* phase, the muscle membrane becomes permeable to sodium ions. A critical threshold is reached. A muscle action potential occurs, which goes in both directions along the muscle fiber. Cells release calcium ions, and muscle contraction occurs.

Next comes the *repolarization* phase. The membrane potential returns to normal. Sodium conduction is blocked. There is a sodium-potassium exchange (like hostages). Now the muscle is ready to be stimulated by another nerve impulse.

Nondepolarizing agents block the receptor sites binding acetylcholine.

Depolarizing agents stimulate and prolong depolarization of postsynaptic receptors.

Q3. In your own words describe the events that occur in depolarization and repolarization.

_____

_____

_____

_____

_____

Nondepolarizing Agents

Nondepolarizing agents get their name because stimulation and depolarization of the muscle never occur.

Mode of Action
Nondepolarizing drugs act by competitive inhibition—like a big bully. Their effect is dose related. Larger doses block more receptors. This blockade could be reversed by making more acetylcholine available to compete for receptor sites.

Pharmacokinetics
Q4. The IV route is usually used because it provides _____ onset for neuromuscular blockade—actually within 1 to 2 minutes.

Here's what happens (it's not pretty):

1. Hazy vision
2. Relaxed jaw
3. Drooping eyelids
4. Inability to raise head
5. Paralysis of legs, arms, and finally diaphragm, in that order

Maximal paralyzing effect is reached within 2 to 10 minutes. Are you picturing the poor bison who's been shot by a poison dart? Are there bison in South America? Anyway.

Q5. Recovery is in reverse order, so which function returns first? _____

Q6. Last? _____

Duration of action is fairly long (around 35 to 60 minutes), and complete recovery may take several hours.

Metabolism
Tubocurarine and metocurine are not metabolized. With these drugs 50% to 60% of the dose is excreted in the urine.

Hazards and Adverse Effects
Cardiovascular:

- Tachycardia
- Increased mean arterial pressure (MAP)

These side effects are caused by tubocurarine and pancuronium. The newer drugs in this category (vecuronium, atracurium, pipecuronium) have minimal effects on heart rate or blood pressure.

Histamine release:

All nondepolarizing agents provoke histamine release from mast cells, but the degree of effect depends on the drug. Tubocurarine causes the greatest release of histamine, which may cause bronchospasm and increased airway resistance.

Q7. Why is this bad? _____

_____

_____

Q8. Pancuronium and vecuronium don't provoke much release of histamines, so they might be better choices, especially in which patients?

_____

Inadequate ventilation:

Muscle paralysis (the diaphragm is not spared) results in apnea—duh. So while the patient is paralyzed, you must support his or her ventilation. I feel as if I have just insulted your intelligence—sorry.

Reversal of Nondepolarizing Blockade

This can be accomplished by the following:

- Use of cholinesterase inhibitors

OR

- Indirect-acting parasympathomimetics

Nondepolarizing Blocking Agents

Examples of nondepolarizing blocking agents include physostigmine, neostigmine, pyridostigmine, and edrophonium.

Depolarizing Agents

Depolarizing agents have a different mode of action from nondepolarizing agents, are much shorter acting, and have no antidote for reversing the blockade. Muscle paralysis will occur in 1 to 1.5 minutes and last from 10 to 15 minutes. Succinylcholine is the only agent in this group.

Mode of Action

Initial muscle contraction occurs, followed by flaccid paralysis. Vagal ganglia stimulation occurs, causing bradycardia and hypotension. Then sympathetic ganglia stimulation occurs, which leads to transient hypertension and tachycardia. Succinylcholine also causes histamine release.

Reversal

Can't be done. You just have to wait until it wears off.

Hazards and Adverse Effects

- Muscle soreness
- Increased serum potassium level—Succinylcholine causes an efflux of potassium from cells. This is bad because hyperkalemia can cause cardiac dysrhythmias or arrest.
- Increased intracranial pressure—This is bad for patients with head trauma or cerebral edema.

Use with Mechanical Ventilation

Neuromuscular blocking agents are typically used in patients who are not breathing in rhythm with the ventilator, who are "fighting" the ventilator. This causes the patient's work of breathing to increase (not good). The goal of using neuromuscular blocking agents is to improve gas exchange, decrease the patient's work of breathing, and reduce ventilating pressures.

Precautions and Risks

When patients are paralyzed, they are usually frightened and anxious. (Wouldn't you be?) Therefore the patients should be sedated and receive pain control.

When a patient is paralyzed, you can't rely on clinical signs (like restlessness or anxiety) to tell you when there's a problem. Close cardiac and ventilatory monitoring becomes that much more important. Tachycardia may be an indication of anxiety (caused by inadequate sedation or pain control) or clinical deterioration, the treatments for which are very different.

Patients who are paralyzed for extended periods of time may need physical therapy (range of motion exercises) to lessen the potential for muscle atrophy.

Q9. What implication do weak respiratory muscles have on ventilator weaning?

_____

_____

Choice of Agents

How do you decide which neuromuscular agent to use? Obviously, it depends. Succinylcholine (depolarizing) is good for intubation because it acts quickly and doesn't last long. Nondepolarizing agents are better for long-term ventilator use. Another plus with nondepolarizing agents is the fact that they can be reversed with cholinesterase inhibitors, like neostigmine.

Keep in mind that even though all nondepolarizing agents cause histamine release, some are worse than others. Pancuronium has the lowest amount.

Q 10. Pancuronium would be a good choice for which patients? _____

Vecuronium has minimal effects on the cardiovascular system (heart rate, blood pressure), so if you have a patient who is a little unstable (in the cardiovascular sense, of course), vecuronium is a good choice. Vecuronium also causes a minimal amount of histamine release, so it's a good overall choice.

Q 11. The preferred route of administration is _____, to adjust the dose easily and provide rapid and complete onset.

Interaction with Antibiotics
The following antibiotics can cause neuromuscular blockade as a side effect. Eek!

- Aminoglycosides (like gentamicin)
- Tetracyclines
- Lincomycin
- Polymyxins
- Clindamycin

Use of Sedatives and Analgesics
Q 12. Remember that although neuromuscular blocking agents cause _____, they do not affect consciousness. It is absolutely necessary to provide sedation and pain control for patients who are paralyzed! The most commonly used drugs for sedation of ventilator patients are morphine sulfate, lorazepam, and diazepam (Valium), in that order.

Monitoring
You can assess the degree of paralysis and/or return of muscle function by the following:

- Hand grip strength
- Negative inspiratory force
- Vital capacity
- Ability to hold head up for 5 seconds

Q 13. When you're ready to wean the patient from the ventilator, _____ the level of sedation and muscle paralysis.

Here they are.

1. Neuromuscular blocking agents are used for all but which of the following?
   a. Endotracheal extubation
   b. Muscle paralysis during surgery
   c. To facilitate mechanical ventilation
   d. Endotracheal intubation
   (Chapter 18, p. 294)

2. If a mechanically ventilated patient is receiving vecuronium, the patient should also receive which of the following?
   a. Sedation
   b. Analgesics
   c. Physical therapy
   d. All the above
   (Chapter 18, pp. 300-301)

3. Muscle contraction occurs during which of the following?
   a. Apolarization
   b. Depolarization
   c. Repolarization
   d. Myelination   (Chapter 18, p. 295)

4. The only depolarizing drug is which of the following?
   a. Tubocurarine
   b. Doxacurium
   c. Pancuronium
   d. Succinylcholine   (Chapter 18, p. 298)

5. Nondepolarizing agents prevent the occurrence of which of the following?
   I. Muscle contraction
   II. Muscle relaxation
   III. Depolarization
   IV. Repolarization

   a. I and III
   b. I and IV
   c. II and III
   d. II and IV   (Chapter 18, p. 295)

6. The preferred route of administration for neuromuscular blocking agents is which of the following?
   a. IM
   b. Oral
   c. Aerosol
   d. IV   (Chapter 18, p. 294)

7. Which is paralyzed first when a nondepolarizing agent is used?
   a. Diaphragm
   b. Arms
   c. Legs
   d. a and b   (Chapter 18, p. 296)

8. Tubocurarine accomplishes which of the following?
   a. Causes stabilization of mast cells
   b. Causes hypotension
   c. Causes tachycardia
   d. Causes the least amount of histamine release   (Chapter 18, p. 297)

9. Muscle paralysis caused by nondepolarizing blocking agents can be reversed by which of the following?
   a. Cholinesterase
   b. Cholinesterase inhibitors
   c. Parasympatholytics
   d. Sympathomimetics
                    (Chapter 18, p. 297)

10. Which of the following describes succinylcholine?
    a. Is long-acting
    b. Cannot by reversed
    c. Does not produce histamine release
    d. May cause sodium retention
                    (Chapter 18, pp. 298-299)

Sim

You are staffing the emergency department. A motor vehicle accident victim is being brought in. He is believed to have pulmonary contusion and flail chest. He does not respond to verbal commands and is combative. Based on his arterial blood gases, the physician has decided to let you intubate the patient. The patient is very restless. Which neuromuscular blocking agent should you use to paralyze him? Why?

_____
_____
_____

Answer: Succinylcholine is a good choice because it takes effect quickly and wears off in 10 to 15 minutes. This will give you enough time to intubate and stabilize the endotracheal tube without leaving him paralyzed unnecessarily long.

He is moved to the ICU on your shift. When you come back the next day, he is breathing asynchronously with the vent. Which type of blocking agent do you recommend? Why?

_____
_____
_____

Answer: Use a nondepolarizing agent for long-term ventilator care. Vecuronium is a good choice because it has minimal effects on both the cardiovascular system and histamine release. Don't forget to see that your patient is provided with sedation, pain control, and physical therapy.

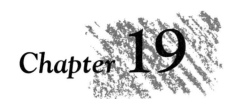

Chapter 19 Cardiac Drugs

Basically, cardiac drugs are divided into two groups: those used to stimulate the heart and those used to regulate dysrhythmias.

Cardiovascular System

The whole cardiovascular system functions as an interdependent set of components. Here's what it looks like:

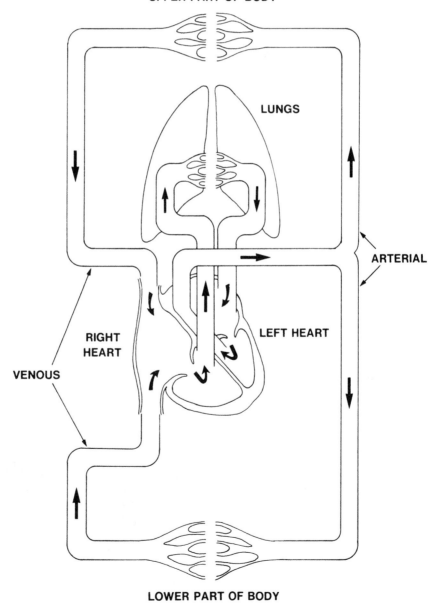

UPPER PART OF BODY

LUNGS

ARTERIAL

RIGHT
HEART

LEFT HEART

VENOUS

LOWER PART OF BODY

Refer back to this illustration when you're learning about which drugs affect which part of the system or how changes in one part can affect the rest of the system.

Factors Affecting Blood Pressure

Blood pressure, specifically MAP, shows how the cardiovascular system is interrelated:

MAP = Cardiac output × Total peripheral resistance

Q 1. Resistance to blood flow depends on viscosity and to a greater extent vessel radius. So vasoconstrictors _____ the size of the vessel, so they _____ resistance. The relationship is inverse.

Cardiac output depends on blood volume, venous return, and contractile force of the heart. Fill in the blanks with the word *increase* or *decrease*.

Q 2. Increased blood volume will _____ cardiac output.

Q 3. Decreased venous return will _____ cardiac output.

Q 4. Increased contractile force will _____ cardiac output.

The whole point of having an adequate blood pressure (arterial perfusion) is to adequately perfuse and oxygenate the tissues. In general, cardiac drugs, whatever the type, are developed to produce an adequate cardiac output. We'll look at the resistance aspect in Chapter 20—vasodilators and vasoconstrictors. (Can you stand to wait?)

Heart

Look at the figure below. It shows the main cardiac events in a normal heartbeat and their corresponding electrical counterparts seen on ECG. The four major areas of the heart important for cardiac drugs are sinoatrial (SA) node, atrial muscle, atrioventricular (AV) node, and ventricular muscle.

Normally, an electrical signal arises from the SA node, resulting in an ECG tracing with a P wave, QRS complex, and T wave.

Action Potentials

The action potential of myocardial cells is divided into five phases:

Phase 0—rapid depolarization with rapid inward flow of sodium ions ("fast response")

Phase 1—early, incomplete repolarization

Phase 2—influx of calcium ions ("slow response"). Depolarizing action of calcium influx overlaps with the repolarizing action of the sodium pump.

Phase 3—rapid repolarization

Phase 4—resting state

Basic Dysrhythmias

Normal cardiac function requires an adequate force of contraction (resulting from the electrical depolarization recorded on the ECG).

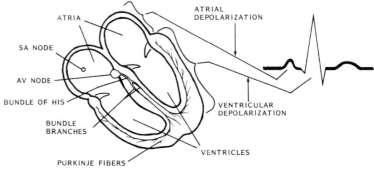

Failure to mechanically pump blood *with* the presence of electrical activity is called EMD (electromechanical dissociation).

The basic cardiac dysrhythmias you'll see on an ECG and for which cardiac drugs will be used include bradycardia, tachycardias, premature beats, atrial and ventricular fibrillation, asystole, and degrees of heart conduction block.

Because the heart requires oxygen just like any other organ, the way in which oxygen consumption is affected by various cardiac drugs is important to consider.

Terminology of Cardiac and Cardiovascular Agents

If you don't know the following terms, you'll be lost later:

Chronotropic—rate of cardiac contraction (heart rate less than 40 or higher than 140 beats/min lower cardiac output)

Inotropic—force of cardiac contraction

Preload—tension on the cardiac muscle as it begins to contract. This is measured as the volume of blood in the ventricle immediately before contraction (systole). The more the ventricular fibers stretch to accommodate more volume, the harder the heart will have to work.

Afterload—amount of resistance against which the heart must pump

Q 5. What effect might preload and afterload have on cardiat output? Explain it in your own words.

_____

_____

_____

_____

Central Venous and Pulmonary Artery Wedge Pressure

Central venous pressure (CVP) gives an estimate of filling pressure in the right ventricle.

Normal is 0 to 6 mm Hg. Pulmonary artery wedge pressure (PAWP) gives an indication of filling pressure in the left ventricle. Normal is 6 to 12 mm Hg. An easy way to estimate how various conditions will affect these parameters is to remember the following:

Volume = Pressure

Try this out. Patient 1 has left ventricular failure. His heart won't pump very well, his ventricle is dilated, and the blood just pools in there because his heart can't beat strong enough to remove it all. What is his PAWP? (High, low, or normal?)

Answer: Volume = Pressure

He's got increased volume, so PAWP is high.

Would this patient benefit from a chronotropic or an inotropic drug? _____

Answer: Assuming that the patient isn't all that far gone, an inotropic drug would be of most benefit to him because it increases the force of contraction. An increased heart rate won't do him any good.

Cardiotonic (Positive Inotropic) Drugs

Cardiac Glycosides

Digitalis is the dried leaf of the foxglove plant, *Digitalis purpurea*. The term *digitalis* is used to refer to the whole group of related drugs called glycosides.

Q 6. The main effect of glycosides on the myocardium is to increase the strength of contraction, a positive _____ effect.

Digitoxin is the longest acting; digoxin (Lanoxin) is intermediate in onset and duration

Q 7. Would you choose digitoxin or digoxin for use in the acute care setting? _____

Mode of Action
Glycosides work by inactivating the sodium pump, causing an increase in intracellular sodium and calcium. Calcium promotes an increased force of contraction (positive inotropic effect.). Heart rate decreases because of vagal stimulation and impaired AV conduction.

Clinical Use
•CHF (cardiotonic) •Atrial flutter or fibrillation (antiarrhythmic)

The cardiotonic effect increases cardiac output, decreases heart size and CVP, and improves diuresis.

*Q*8. What does CVP indicate? _____

The antiarrhythmic effect is caused by slowing AV conduction.

Phosphodiesterase Inhibitors
Amrinone and milrinone are examples of phosphodiesterase inhibitors. They have both positive inotropic and vasodilating effects, so they are used to increase cardiac output. Preload and afterload are both reduced by the relaxation of vascular smooth muscle.

*Q*9. In patients with CHF, phosphodiesterase inhibitors are used to _____ cardiac output, _____ systemic vascular resistance (SVR), and improve left ventricular function.

*Q*10. Remember, volume equals pressure. So if my preload decreases, what effect should that have on my PAWP?

_____

It's not fully understood how these drugs work, but they are selective for phosphodiesterase enzymes in cardiac and vascular smooth muscle. When phosphodiesterase is inhibited, cyclic AMP is increased, myocardial contractility is increased, and blood vessels are dilated.

Beta-Adrenergic Cardiac Stimulants
Agents that stimulate beta-1 adrenergic receptors can increase heart rate and contractility, thus increasing cardiac output.

Epinephrine
*Q*11. Epinephrine is a catecholamine, stimulating both alpha and beta receptors. It increases both heart rate and strength of contraction, _____ cardiac output.

*Q*12. Alpha stimulation (vasoconstriction) can also increase blood pressure; beta-2 stimulation can cause _____

Epinephrine is used to treat asystole or fine ventricular fibrillation (before elecrical countershock).

Isoproterenol
Does isoproterenol sound familiar? This was also mentioned before as a bronchodilator.

*Q*13. Isoproterenol is not very selective for beta-2 stimulation, so beta-1 receptors are also stimulated, causing increased _____ and _____.

But increased cardiac output causes increased myocardial oxygen consumption, which can cause extended infarction (not good).

Isoproterenol is used for emergency control of severe bradycardia (vvveeerrryyy ssslllooowww) that doesn't respond to atropine.

Dobutamine (Dobutrex)
Dobutamine is a synthetic catecholamine, whose primary effect is as a beta-1 stimulant.

*Q*14. Dobutamine's cardiovascular effect is inotropic, meaning an increase in

_____.

$\mathcal{Q}$15. Dobutamine is a wonder because it doesn't increase total peripheral resistance, so it can _____ cardiac output without increasing blood pressure, afterload, and myocardial work.

Dobutamine is given IV for CHF and with nitroprusside after cardiopulmonary bypass surgery to recover cardiovascular status.

Antiarrhythmic Agents

There are four classes of antiarrhythmic agents:

Class I
Class I agents are membrane-stabilizing or local anesthetics that depress the fast inward current of sodium (phase 0). Examples include the following:

- Quinidine—used for atrial fibrillation and flutter, paroxysmal atrial tachycardia (PAT), ventricular tachycardia, and premature ventricular contractions (PVCs)
- Procainamide—used to treat ventricular ectopic beats, ventricular tachycardia, and atrial arrhythmias
- Lidocaine—used to control PVCs, ventricular tachycardia, and ventricular fibrillation

Class II
Class II agents are beta-adrenergic blocking agents. They block beta-1 receptors in the heart to control dysrhythmias. Heart rate is reduced, AV conduction is prolonged, and contractile force is decreased. Lots of class II agents are used to control hypertension.

Examples include the following:

- Propranolol and esmolol—slow supraventricular tachycardias

Class III
Class III agents prolong the duration of phase 3 repolarization and therefore the effective refractory period (increases the action potential).

$\mathcal{Q}$16. Look back a few pages and define action potential. _____

Examples include the following:
- Bretylium—used to treat ventricular tachycardia and fibrillation, resistant to defibrillation, epinephrine, and lidocaine
- Amiodarone—used for recurrent ventricular fibrillation and hemodynamically unstable ventricular tachycardia

Class IV
Class IV agents inhibit the slow channel influx of calcium, in both pacemaker and myocardial cells; coronary artery vasodilation; and treatment of hypertension. These drugs are called calcium channel blockers. Examples include the following:

- Verapamil and diltiazem—used to treat supraventricular tachycardias

$\mathcal{Q}$17. Okay, I'll give you a drug, you list the class. When you list the class, tell what it's used to treat. Here goes!

	Class	Use
1. Propranolol	_____	
2. Verapamil	_____	
3. Quinidine	_____	
4. Lidocaine	_____	

Other Antiarrhythmic Agents

Calcium Chloride
Calcium chloride provides calcium ions necessary for the heart to contract. Calcium ions increase the force of contraction, producing an effect sort of like digitalis.

Q 18. Calcium chloride is used to reverse electromechanical dissociation (EMD). Do you remember what this is? I didn't think so. Look back and write the definition. _____

_____

It also increases cardiac output.

Atropine

Remember when we talked about atropine as a bronchodilator? Well, atropine blocks vagal slowing of the SA and AV nodes. (It blocks decreased heart rate.) So heart rate increases.

Magnesium

Cardiac muscle needs magnesium to repolarize. Low magnesium can also inhibit replenishment of intracellular potassium (which may cause cardiac dysrhythmias). Magnesium supplementation is used to correct hypomagnesemia in refractory ventricular tachycardia and fibrillation.

Potassium

Potassium is also critical to repolarization. Either too much or not enough can cause serious dysrhythmias, so normalization of potassium levels is important!

Drugs Used in Advanced Cardiac Life Support

The table below summarizes drugs used in advanced cardiac life support (ACLS). Each drug is accompanied by indications for its use and a classification. The classification system is as follows:

Class I—definitely helpful

Class II—acceptable, probably helpful

Class III—acceptable, possibly helpful

Class IV—not indicated, may be harmful

To the questions!

1. MAP =:
   a. Cardiac output × SVR
   b. SVR/ PVR
   c. Cardiac output × Total peripheral resistance
   c. SVR × Total peripheral resistance
      (Chapter 19, p. 305)

2. As vessel size decreases, blood pressure does which of the following?
   a. Increases
   b. Decreases
   c. Remains the same
   d. Blood pressure and vessel size are unrelated (Chapter 19, p. 305)

3. The goal(s) of adequate arterial pressure is/are which of the following?
   a. Increased cardiac output
   b. Tissue perfusion
   c. Tissue oxygenation
   d. b and c (Chapter 19, p. 305)

4. In the heart the pacemaker signal arises spontaneously from which of the following:
   a. SA node
   b. AV node
   c. Purkinje fibers
   d. Branch bundles (Chapter 19, p. 307)

5. Which phase of the heart's action potential is synonymous with diastole (relaxation)?
   a. 1
   b. 2
   c. 3
   d. 4 (Chapter 19, p. 308)

6. Failure of the heart to mechanically pump blood with the presence of electrical activity is which of the following?
   a. Bradycardia
   b. Dysystole
   c. EMD
   d. WGD (Chapter 19, p. 308)

Drug or group	Use/ECC-AHA recommendation
Lidocaine	VT, VF after defibrillation and epinephrine; or ventricular ectopy, or wide-complex PSVT (class I); prophylactic therapy to prevent VF after acute MI with no PVCs (class IIb)
Procainamide	PVCs and recurrent VT if lidocaine fails/contraindicated (class IIa)
Bretylium	Resistant VT/VF unresponsive to defibrillation, epinephrine, lidocaine (class IIa)
Beta-adrenergic blockers (atenolol, metoprolol, propranolol)	May reduce rate of recurrent MI in thrombolytic-treated patients (not recommended routinely); used to reduce incidence of VF after MI if thrombolytic therapy not used (recommended)
Atropine	Symptomatic sinus bradycardia (class I); for AV block at nodal level (class IIa) or ventricular asystole
Isoproterenol	Refractory torsades de pointes, acute temporary control of bradycardia in denervated hearts of transplant recipients (class IIa)
Verapamil/diltiazem	To control ventricular rates in narrow-complex PSVT (second to adenosine) if reentrant arrhythmia involving AV node; or for rate control in atrial fibrillation
Adenosine	To terminate PSVT involving a reentry pathway including the AV node (recommended)

AHA, American Heart Association; AV, atrioventricular; ECC, Emergency Cardiac Care Committee; MI, myocardial infarction; PSVT, paroxysmal supraventricular tachycardia; PVC, premature ventricular contraction; VT/VF, ventricular tachycardia, fibrillation.

7. Which of the following heart rates (in beats per minute) will decrease cardiac output?
   I. 39
   II. 49
   III. 130
   IV. 145
   a. I, II, III, IV
   b. I and II
   c. I and IV
   d. II and III   (Chapter 19, p. 308)

8. What is the effect of increased afterload on cardiac output?
   a. Cardiac output increases.
   b. Cardiac output decreases.
   c. One will not affect the other.
   d. Asystole occurs.
                          (Chapter 19, p. 309)

9. Which of the following is the main effect of digitalis?
   a. Positive chronotropic
   b. Negative chronotropic
   c. Positive inotropic
   d. Negative inotropic
   (Chapter 19, p. 310)

10. Lidocaine is used to control which of the following?
    a. Atrial dysrhythmias
    b. Ventricular dysrhythmias
    c. Heart block
    d. b and c   (Chapter 19, p. 313)

Sim

Your CCU patient suffers from CHF. Her CVP is 20 mm Hg. Is this anything to be concerned about? _____

Answer: Please! It's really high! Normal is less than 6 mm Hg.

Her right ventricle is dilated, and she needs a positive inotropic drug to pump out that blood! Look back through the drugs listed in the "Cardiotonic Drug" section. What would you give her? Why? What effects will the drug have on her CHF?

_____
_____
_____
_____
_____

Answer: You could have chosen digitalis (positive inotrope, increases cardiac output, decreases heart size and CVP); phosphodiesterase inhibitors (positive inotrope, reduces preload and afterload, decreases PAWP, increases cardiac output); dobutamine (positive inotrope, increases cardiac output without increased afterload).

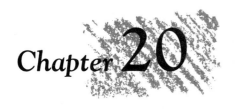

Chapter 20 Drugs Affecting Circulation

There are four important classes of drugs that affect the circulatory system. We'll discuss them in this chapter, but first, let's review the circulatory system and hypertension.

Circulatory System

What's the purpose of the circulatory system?

_____

_____

If you said that it's to supply oxygenated blood to the tissues, you're right!

When coronary arteries are obstructed, there's not enough blood flow to the myocardium. This ischemia results in angina and may ultimately cause infarction, heart failure, or even cardiac arrest, which means the tissues get inadequate or no perfusion.

Q1. Patients in shock have excessively low arterial pressures, leading to _____ perfusion pressure for blood supply to the tissues.

Hypertension and Treatment

Adult hypertension is defined as a blood pressure equal to or higher than 140/90 mm Hg. There are many drugs available to treat hypertension (diuretics, antiadrenergic, beta-adrenergic blockade, vasodilators, etc.).

If there is no primary disorder, high blood pressure is called *essential hypertension*. Treatment of essential hypertension follows a stepped approach, using a selection of drugs that we'll discuss in this chapter.

Antihypertensive Drug Classes

Diuretics
Diuretics work because they increase sodium loss and have a direct effect on blood vessels, thus lowering vascular resistance. Reduction of plasma volume, which will lower blood pressure, isn't maintained with long-term administration of the diuretic. Examples are the thiazides and furosemide.

Centrally Acting Antiadrenergics
Centrally acting antiadrenergic agents are alpha-2 sympathetic agonists. (They are inhibitory.) These drugs act by inhibiting the cardioaccelerator and vasoconstrictor centers. Long-term therapy keeps peripheral resistance low, allowing cardiac output to return to pretreatment values. Examples are methyldopa and clonidine.

Peripherally Acting Antiadrenergic Agents
Q2. Peripherally acting antiadrenergic agents inhibit the release of norepinephrine, causing a relaxation of vascular smooth muscle, decreased total vascular resistance, and _____ blood pressure. Drugs in this category include guanethidine and prazosin.

Classes of Antihypertensive Agents, with Representative Agents

Diuretics
  thiazides
  furosemide
  amiloride
  spironolactone
  triamterene

Antiadrenergic—Central Activity
  methyldopa (Aldomet)
  clonidine (Catapres)
  guanabenz (Wytensin)
  guanfacine (Tenex)

Antiadrenergic—Peripheral Activity
  reserpine (Serpasil)
  guanethidine (Ismelin)
  guanadrel (Hylorel)
  doxazosin (Cardura)
  prazosin (Minipress)
  terazosin (Hytrin)

Beta-adrenergic Blockade
  acebutolol (Sectral)
  atenolol (Tenormin)
  betaxolol (Kerlone)
  bisoprolol (Zebeta)
  carteolol (Cartrol)
  metoprolol (Lopressor)
  nadolol (Corgard)
  penbutolol (Levatol)
  pindolol (Visken)
  propranolol (Inderal)
  timolol (Blocadren)

Alpha- and Beta-Adrenergic Blockade
  labetalol (Normodyne, Trandate)

Vasodilation—Direct Acting
  hydralazine (Apresoline)
  minoxidil (Loniten)

Angiotensin Converting Enzyme (ACE) Inhibition
  benazepril (Lotensin)
  captopril (Capoten)
  enalapril (Vasotec)
  fosinopril (Monopril)
  lisinopril (Prinivil)
  moexipril hydrochloride (Univasc)
  quinapril (Accupril)
  ramipril (Altace)
  trandolapril (Mavik)

Angiotensin II Antagonist
  losartan potassium (Cozaar)
  valsartan (Diovan)

Calcium Channel Blocking Agents
  amlodipine (Norvasc)
  diltiazem (Cardizem)
  felodipine (Plendil)
  isradipine (DynaCirc)
  nicardipine (Cardene)
  verapamil (Calan, Isoptin)

Emergency (Acute) Antihypertensives
  nitroprusside (Nipride)
  diazoxide (Hyperstat)
  nitroglycerin IV

Miscellaneous Agents
  mecamylamine (Inversine)
  pargyline

Agents for Pheochromocytoma
  phentolamine (Regitine)
  phenoxybenzamine hydrochloride (Dibenzyline)
  metyrosine (Demser)

Beta-Adrenergic Blockade

Q3. Beta-adrenergic blockers block beta-1 receptors in the _____. Both chronotropic and inotropic responses to beta-adrenergic stimulation are blocked. Cardiac output decreases, and so does blood pressure. Examples include acebutolol and propranolol.

Alpha- and Beta-Adrenergic Blockade

Q4. Guess what? Alpha- and beta-adrenergic blockers block _____ and _____ receptors, hence, the name! This class basically works using a combination of the preceding groups of drugs. An example of this classification is labetalol.

Vasodilators

Nitroglycerin is probably the best-known example of a vasodilator. Vasodilators lower blood pressure by a direct relaxation of vascular smooth muscle. Minoxidil (you thought it was only for bald people with hypertension!) and hydralazine are other examples.

Angiotensin Converting Enzyme Inhibition

Angiotensin converting enzyme (ACE) inhibitors act by interfering with the system that produces angiotensin II. Angiotensin II causes secretion of aldosterone. Aldosterone causes sodium retention and increased blood pressure.

Q5. So because ACE inhibitors interfere with that whole sequence of events, blood pressure _____.

ACE inhibitors are contraindicated in pregnancy. They can cause injury or death to the fetus if used during the second or third trimesters. Benazepril and captopril are examples of ACE inhibitors.

Acute Antihypertensive Agents

Sodium nitroprusside has a direct action on peripheral blood vessels, causing vasodilation on both venous and arterial circulation. The effects of these drugs begin rapidly with IV administration and end when infusion is stopped. Nitroprusside (Nipride) and nitroglycerin are emergency antihypertensive agents.

Antianginal Agents

Antianginal agents are primarily used to treat (you guessed it!) angina pectoris! Angina is a paroxysmal precordial pain, with a feeling of suffocation. Angina may be triggered by exertion or excitement in coronary artery disease.

6. Angina is caused by decreased blood flow to the heart muscle, which has what effect on the oxygen demands of the heart? _____

There are three classes of drugs to treat angina. As luck would have it, we'll cover all three! Each class accomplishes one of the following:

- Decreases peripheral vascular resistance
- Decreases cardiac output
- OR Both

Nitrates and Nitrites

The class consisting of nitrates and nitrites is used to relieve anginal pain. They're systemic vasodilators. They work by increasing nitric oxide in vascular smooth muscle tissue. Nitric oxide stimulates guanyl cyclase to produce cyclic GMP, decreased intracellular calcium, and smooth muscle relaxation. Nitroglycerin is the best known of the nitrates. It's available via IV, sublingual tablet, translingual spray, transmucosal tablet, topical ointment, transdermal pad, oral tablets, and capsules.

Calcium Channel Blockers

*Q*7. We've already talked about calcium channel blockers as _____ and antihypertensive agents, but they're also used to treat angina. Calcium channels are blocked, calcium influx decreases, smooth muscle relaxes, myocardial contractility is reduced, and cardiac output is decreased. These drugs are used if nitrates or beta blockers aren't well tolerated. You've also got to be careful about hypotension brought on by all that relaxation and slowing down of the heart!

Beta-Adrenergic Blocking Agents

*Q*8. Beta-adrenergic blocking agents block cardiac beta-_____ receptors! Heart rate decreases, cardiac output decreases, blood pressure falls, and myocardial oxygen demand is reduced.

*Q*9. Complete the table below with yes or no:

Class	Decreased vascular resistance	Decreased cardiac output
Nitrates and nitrites		
Calcium channel blockers		
Beta-adrenergic blockers		

Vasoconstricting Agents (Vasopressors)

Vasopressors are used to treat shock (caused by inadequate tissue perfusion). The box above lists several types of shock and the corresponding cause.

Types and Causes of Shock	
Type	**Cause**
hypovolemic	fluid loss
cardiogenic	cardiac dysfunction
septic	septicemia
blood flow obstruction	embolus, aneurysm
neurogenic	spinal injury or drug induced
anaphylactic	hypersensitivity reaction

The primary goal of vasopressor therapy is to support blood pressure until the underlying cause of shock is reversed. There are two ways to increase blood pressure: positive inotropism and vasoconstriction. The table on the next page lists the pharmacological agents used to treat shock along with their sites of action and hemodynamic response.

Antithrombotic Drug Classes

Let's get a few terms straight.

Embolism—obstruction of a blood vessel by a foreign object, like a clot, fat, or air

Thrombus—blood clot that obstructs a vessel or cavity of the heart

Thromboembolism—blocking of a blood vessel by a thrombus that has become detached from its site of formation (a moving clot)

Damage to a blood vessel results in immediate vasospasm to limit bleeding. Collagen is exposed to the blood. Collagen attracts and binds platelets. Platelets stick to each other, forming a platelet plug to limit bleeding at the damaged site. Clotting factors are activated. A fibrin clot is formed.

Pharmacological Agents Used in Treating Shock, with Their Sites of Action and Hemodynamic Responses

The spectrum of activity shifts from the positive inotropes at the top of the table, to the pure vasoconstrictors in the bottom rows.

	Cardiac Contractility	Vasoconstriction	Vasodilation	Cardiac Output	Peripheral Resistance
Isoproterenol	+++	O	+++	⇑	⇓
Dobutamine	+++	O/+	+	⇑	⇓
Dopamine	+++	+ to +++*	O/+†	⇑	⇕*
Epinephrine	+++	+++*	++*	⇑	⇓
Norepinephrine	++	+++	O	O/⇓	⇑
Ephedrine	++	+	O/+	⇑	⇕
Mephentermine	+	+	++	⇑	O/⇑
Metaraminol	+	++	O	⇓	⇑
Methoxamine	O	+++	O	O/⇓	⇑
Phenylephrine	O	+++	O	⇑⇓	

Based on data in *Facts and comparisons*, St Louis, 1997, JB Lippincott.

*Effect is dose dependent and/or receptor type (alpha, beta-2) dependent.

†Dilates renal, splanchnic vessels at lower doses.

There are proteins in plasma that limit the spread of clotting from the injury site, so your body just doesn't go wild, clotting all over the place. This can happen, though, if those plasma proteins are overwhelmed or missing. Generalized intravascular clotting is called disseminated intravascular coagulation (DIC).

Q 10. There are three classes of drugs used to treat or prevent thrombi. A thrombus is defined as _____.

Anticoagulant Agents
Anticoagulant agents are commonly used in the clinical setting, and include heparin and the coumarin group.

Heparin—binds to antithrombin III, causing a structural change in the antithrombin, which inhibits the conversion (by thrombin) of fibrinogen to fibrin. What?

Q 11. Write it out once in your own words and it will make sense _____.

Heparin is given IV in the acute care setting. It's often given when a patient is at risk for pulmonary embolism following extended bed rest (like after surgery). The major risk of heparin, of course, is bleeding. It's contraindicated in states of active bleeding like (Arkansas)—kidding, hypertension, intracranial hemorrhage, or ulcers. Heparin disappears rapidly from the blood.

The dose of heparin is titrated by monitoring the anticoagulant effect through partial thromboplastin time (PTT), which should be kept around 2 to 2.5 times the normal value. Normal value is 22 to 37 seconds.

Coumarin group—warfarin—given orally and used for chronic treatment of thromboembolic conditions, good for maintenance therapy.

The coumarin group drugs work by preventing the reactivation of vitamin K. There is a delay of up to several days to see the anticoagulant effect with warfarin. The dose is titrated by monitoring the anticoagulant effect through prothrombin time (PT).

Q 12. List one similarity and one difference between heparin and warfarin.

Difference:

_____

Similarity:

_____

Antiplatelet Agents

The classic antiplatelet agent is aspirin, which prevents platelet aggregation. One indication for the use of aspirin (acetylsalicylic acid, ASA) is acute myocardial infarction. An oral dose of 160 mg is given ASAP after the infarct occurs. ASA is also used to treat the following:

- Angina
- Postinfarction follow-up
- Postcoronary artery bypass surgery
- Coronary angioplasty
- Prevention of strokes
- Transient ischemic attacks (TIA)—ministrokes

Who knew all of this was in that little green bottle?

Thrombolytic Agents

Thrombolytic agents cause the conversion of plasminogen to plasmin. Plasmin initiates local fibrinolysis in a blood clot. The following lists two types of thrombolytic agents:

- Tissue plasminogen activators (tPAs) are used in the management of acute myocardial infarction, strokes, and pulmonary embolism.
- Thrombolytic enzymes like *streptokinase* are given IV for acute myocardial infarction, pulmonary embolism, deep vein thrombus, and arterial thrombosis. *Urokinase* is another example, given IV for massive pulmonary embolus or coronary artery thrombosis to prevent myocardial infarction.

Are you wondering when you'll have a chance to test your knowledge on circulatory system drugs? The wait is over.

1. Adult hypertension is defined as blood pressure equal to or higher than which of the following?
   a. 130/75
   b. 140/90
   c. 150/100
   d. 180/120   (Chapter 20, p. 319)

2. Essential hypertension may be treated with which of the following?
   I. Beta blockers
   II. Moderation of alcohol intake
   III. ACE inhibitors
   IV. Regular physical exercise

   a. I, II, III, IV
   b. I and III
   c. II and IV
   d. I, II, IV   (Chapter 20, pp. 319-320)

3. All but which of the following are true of diuretics?
   a. They increase sodium loss.
   b. They reduce plasma volume.
   c. They lower vascular resistance.
   d. They inhibit alpha-2 receptors.
                      (Chapter 20, p. 321)

4. Beta blockers accomplish which of the following?
   a. Block beta-2 receptors in the heart
   b. Stimulate chronotropic response
   c. Decrease blood pressure
   d. Stimulate inotropic response
   (Chapter 20, pp. 322-323)

5. Nitroglycerin is used to treat which of the following?
   a. Angina
   b. Hypertension
   c. Post myocardial infarction
   d. a and b   (Chapter 20, p. 324)

6. Which of the following is paroxysmal precordial pain accompanied by a feeling of suffocation?
   a. Angina pectoris
   b. Shock
   c. Acute myocardial infarction
   d. TIA   (Chapter 20, p. 324)

7. An increased concentration of nitric oxide in vascular smooth muscle causes which of the following?
   a. Vasoconstriction
   b. Bronchoconstriction
   c. Vasodilation
   d. Bronchodilation (Chapter 20, p. 325)

8. Which of the following classes of antianginal drugs decreases both vascular resistance and cardiac output?
   a. nitrates
   b. calcium channel blockers
   c. beta blockers
   d. b and c   (Chapter 20, p. 325)

9. Which of the following describes inadequate tissue perfusion?
   a. Results in shock
   b. Requires vasodilator therapy
   c. Requires blood pressure support
   d. a and c   (Chapter 20, p. 325)

10. Aspirin is classified as which of the following?
    a. Antithrombotic
    b. Anticoagulant
    c. Coumarin
    d. Antiplatelet (Chapter 20, pp. 329-330)

Sim

Your patient is a 43-year-old motor vehicle accident victim who has suffered extensive blood loss and is now in shock. What is "shock," and what type does this patient have?

_____
_____
_____

Answer: Shock is defined as inadequate tissue perfusion. This patient is suffering from hypovolemic shock. He has actually lost blood volume. When there's less blood to make the circulatory rounds, tissue perfusion suffers. Go figure!

How will you treat his condition?

_____
_____
_____

Answer: With shock, you must maintain the patient's blood pressure until the underlying cause of the shock can be reversed. To treat the underlying cause, your patient needs blood transfusions, treatment for internal injuries that may have been sustained in the motor vehicle accident, and supportive care as necessary (airway support, mechanical ventilation, nutritional support, etc.). To treat the low blood pressure, use a vasoconstrictor (vasopressor), like phenylephrine, methoxamine, or metaraminol; or a positive inotrope, like isoproterenol, dobutamine, or dopamine.

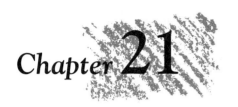

Chapter 21   Diuretic Agents

Diuretics increase urine output. Their main goal in life is to get rid of excess fluid from the body and they act directly on the kidney. Before we look at the diuretics (you knew this was coming), we should review renal function.

Renal Stucture and Function

Normally, how many kidneys does a human have? _____ Yes, two. That's why they're called paired retroperitoneal organs. The kidneys are perfused by the renal artery. Guess what percentage of your cardiac output goes to the renal system? _____ Did you say 21%?

I can't believe you guessed that!

✐1. Circle one. Like the heart and brain, the kidney is (an active organ, a passive filter). This means the kidney has a high oxygen consumption. So if you have circulatory problems, your kidneys are in big trouble!

Functional units of the kidney are called *nephrons*, and each kidney has about a million. You can lose about 75% of your nephrons before you run into problems. The nephron contains the following:

- Glomerulus
- Loop of Henle
- Collecting tubule
- Proximal tubule
- Distal tubule

The glomerulus filters fluid from the blood to the tubule. This fluid empties into the proximal convoluted tubule, goes through the ascending and descending loops of Henle, into the distal convoluted tubule, to the collecting duct, finally emptying into the ureter to be stored in the bladder.

Nephron Function

The nephron has the same ionic concentration as the plasma. In passing through the nephron, more than 99% of the glomerular filtrate is reabsorbed in the tubules. Amazing! This leaves only about 1% to be excreted as urine.

Diuretics interfere, in various ways, with the reabsorption of water in the tubules of the nephron. The amazing nephron does all the following:

- Keeps blood protein and cells out of the glomerular filtrate
- Maintains the alkaline reserve of the blood
- Excretes nitrogenous waste like urea and uric acid
- Eliminates drugs and their breakdown products from the body

The tubules filter and exchange the following:

- Sodium
- Chloride
- Potassium
- Bicarbonate

Acid-Base Balance

Because they increase water loss, diuretics may cause acid-base imbalances. The important exchange for acid-base balance is *sodium*. Sodium gets reabsorbed in the tubules by the following:

- Reabsorption with chloride to preserve electrical neutrality

- Exchange of sodium for hydrogen or potassium (also preserving neutrality)

Low chloride or low potassium will force sodium to exchange for hydrogen. You end up with a net loss of hydrogen ions, which leads to metabolic alkalosis.

Q 2. Soooooo, metabolic alkalosis (a bad thing) can be caused by _____ or _____.

Diuretic Groups

There are five major groups of diuretics. Each group acts at a different site in the nephron. If more than one type of diuretic is used, it can lead to nephron blockade because of all the different sites of action.

Q 3. RCPs and critical care clinicians use diuretics most often to treat heart failure (to reduce circulating volume, _____ preload, and treat symptoms of peripheral edema), and hypertension (to reduce fluid volume).

Osmotic Diuretics
Osmotic diuretics are filtered through the glomerulus but *not* reabsorbed in the tubules. So they carry the osmotic equivalent of water through the nephron for excretion in the urine.

They are used IV to accomplish the following:

- Decrease intraocular pressure
- Decrease intracranial pressure
- Decrease circulatory volume
- Prevent acute renal failure

Examples of osmotic diuretics are urea, mannitol, and glycerin.

Carbonic Anhydrase Inhibitors
Carbonic anhydrase inhibitors act in the proximal tubule, where carbonic anhydrase catalyzes the conversion of CO_2 and H_2O to carbonic acid (H_2CO_3), which dissociates into H^+ and HCO_3^-.

By inhibiting carbonic anhydrase, hydrogen is prevented from being available to exchange for sodium. Both sodium and bicarbonate are lost in the filtrate. The loss of bicarb can cause metabolic acidosis in the blood. The urine will become increasingly alkaline (because of the excreted bicarbonate). Carbonic anhydrase inhibitors are rarely used, but are still used to reduce intraocular pressure in treating glaucoma.

Thiazide Diuretics
Thiazide diuretics work by inhibiting sodium and chloride reabsorption in the distal tubule, with a corresponding loss of water. Depletion of potassium also occurs, which can lead to metabolic alkalosis. These drugs are potent!

This group of diuretics is given orally, and is used to treat CHF and hypertension. After initial therapy, cardiac output normalizes, but peripheral vascular resistance stays low. Examples include benzthiazide, chlorothiazide, and cyclothiazide.

Loop Diuretics
Loop diuretics are really potent and are called "high-ceiling" diuretics. They have a longer peak effect than other groups, and they work by inhibiting the reabsorption of sodium and chloride in the thick ascending limb in the loop of Henle.

Loop diuretics may lead to chloride and/or potassium loss or metabolic alkalosis. Potassium supplements may be necessary.

Use loop diuretics when you need huge amounts of diuresis (like in severe CHF, hepatic cirrhosis, and renal disease)! Furosemide is a famous diuretic in this group.

Potassium-Sparing Diuretics
Based on what we've talked about so far, potassium is usually excreted in the urine in exchange for sodium reabsorption. Potassium-sparing diuretics block sodium reabsorption, which actually decreases the loss of potassium. Potassium is spared, hence, the name. Examples are spironolactone, amiloride, and

triamterene. These diuretics are used to treat edema that doesn't respond to other drugs.

For each of the following diuretic groups, tell whether the most likely problem to result with their use is metabolic alkalosis, metabolic acidosis, or neither.

Q 4. Osmotic diuretics _____

Q 5. Carbonic anhydrase inhibitors _____

Q 6. Thiazide diuretics _____

Q 7. Loop diuretics _____

This chapter was so short, I hope I can come up with 10 questions, so you don't feel cheated!

1. All but which of the following statements are true about diuretics?
   a. Diuretics increase urine output.
   b. Diuretics act directly on the kidney.
   c. Diuretics eliminate excess fluid from the body.
   d. Diuretics are all alike in their mode of action.   (Chapter 21, p. 333)

2. The kidney is which of the following?
   a. Active organ
   b. Passive filter
   c. High oxygen consumer
   d. a and c   (Chapter 21, p. 333)

3. Which of the following are components of the kidney?
   I.   Nephron
   II. Glomerulus
   III. Loop of Henle
   IV. Distal tubule

   a. I, II, III, IV
   b. II, III, IV
   c. I, II, III
   d. I, III, IV   (Chapter 21, p. 333)

4. The functional unit of the kidney is which of the following?
   a. Glomerulus
   b. Tubule
   c. Nephron
   d. Bladder   (Chapter 21, p. 333)

5. The purpose of the nephron is to which of the following?
   a. Maintain the acidic reserve of the blood
   b. Maintain the alkaline reserve of the blood
   c. Maintain waterlike reserve of the blood
   d. Get blood protein to the glomerulus
                        (Chapter 21, p. 334)

6. Which of the following describes osmotic diuretics?
   a. Used to treat CHF
   b. Used to treat chronic renal failure
   c. Used to prevent acute renal failure
   d. a and b   (Chapter 21, p. 336)

7. Carbonic anhydrase inhibitors act in which of the following?
   a. Proximal tubules
   b. Distal tubules
   c. Loop of Henle
   d. Glomerulus   (Chapter 21, p. 337)

8. All but which of the following are true of thiazide diuretics?
   a. They are potent diuretics.
   b. They act in the distal tubule.
   c. They are given orally.
   d. They may cause metabolic acidosis.
                        (Chapter 21, p. 337)

9. Which of the following is true of loop diuretics?
   a. They are relatively weak.
   b. They have a greater peak diuretic effect than other diuretics.
   c. They work in the glomerulus.
   d. a and c   (Chapter 21, pp. 337-338)

10. Potassium-sparing diuretics block which of the following?
    a. Potassium reabsorption
    b. Chloride reabsorption
    c. Bicarbonate reabsorption
    d. Sodium reabsorption
    (Chapter 21, p. 338)

Sim

For this chapter I'll give you a disease state/condition, and you decide which of the five groups of diuretics to use. Use each group only once.

1. hypertension _____

2. edema, resistant to other drugs _____

3. glaucoma _____

4. head trauma _____

5. severe CHF _____

Answer:

1. thiazide diuretics
2. potassium-sparing diuretics
3. carbonic anhydrase inhibitors
4. osmotic diuretics
5. loop diuretics

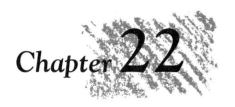

Chapter 22 Drugs Affecting the Central Nervous System

CNS depressants include sedatives, general anesthetics, and psychotherapeutic agents. They can depress the central respiratory centers in the medulla, decreasing the normal response to elevated carbon dioxide levels.

Q 1. By the way, what is the normal response to increased carbon dioxide levels?

_____

If you said hyperventilation, you're a genius. Anyway, if that response is blunted you get hypoventilation or in extreme cases apnea. Overdose of CNS depressants is common in suicide attempts. If a patient is hypoventilating or apneic, what is your job?

Q 2. To support _____.

On the other end of the spectrum, CNS stimulants can cause ventilatory stimulation. Go figure! Here it comes—the review of the CNS.

Central Nervous System

The CNS is functionally divided into the brain and spinal cord. The spinal cord has nerve fibers that transmit information toward the brain and then, from the brain to all areas of the body. Take a look at the brain. It has three parts—the cortex, midbrain, and brain stem.

Cortex
The cortex is a thin layer of cells that covers the whole brain and is responsible for the integration of all bodily functions. It's subdivided into specific areas responsible for different functions, like skeletal muscle control, memory, and intellect. When cortical activity is suppressed by drugs (alcohol is one example), symptoms produce sedation, decreased mental functioning, and slower reflexes.

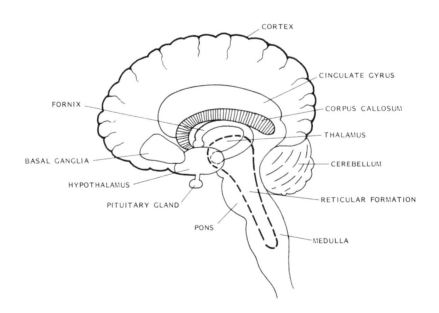

Midbrain

The midbrain contains the thalamus and the hypothalamus. The thalamus is a relay system that sends info from one area of the brain to another and from peripheral sites to the cortex.

  $\mathcal{Q}$3. If a drug suppresses the thalamus, what happens to the speed at which those messages are relayed? _____

The hypothalamus integrates functions of the autonomic nervous system, and controls endocrine function, appetite, and plasma glucose levels.

Medulla

The medulla is the primary structure of the brain stem. It's responsible for maintaining blood pressure and ventilation. Depression of the medulla is a bad thing. If ventilation and the cardiovascular center collapse, what will happen? _____ Yes, death (not good).

Reticular Activating System

The reticular activating system (RAS) is located in the midbrain and serves the following two purposes:

- Stimulation of the cortex to keep you awake (I hope it's working now!)
- Filtering of extraneous sensory info, enhancing your ability to concentrate

If you get bad grades, tell your parents that your RAS is on the blink. The RAS is what allows you to study, even though your roommate is blasting the stereo.

The RAS also mediates the neurogenic drive state that regulates ventilation in response to variations in emotion and activity levels.

  $\mathcal{Q}$4. So when you're asleep and the RAS is not being stimulated much, respiratory rate (increases, decreases).

Limbic System

The limbic system forms a ring around the brain stem and is involved with the control and display of emotion. An abnormality of the limbic system leads to affective disorders like schizophrenia, depression, or manic-depression.

Extrapyramidal System

The structures of the extrapyramidal system are responsible for the control of coordinated fine muscle movement. For example, the cerebellum is responsible for balance.

Central Nervous System Drugs and Sleep State

Drugs that affect CNS function do so in a dose-related fashion and usually in a descending manner, from cortex to brain stem to spinal cord.

  $\mathcal{Q}$5. So small doses may only affect the _____ producing only sedation; large doses may depress the medulla, _____ respiratory and cardiovascular function, leading to _____.

Obviously, sleep is required. The time spent in sleep is divided into slow-wave sleep (SWS) and rapid–eye movement (REM) sleep. SWS is necessary to overcome physical fatigue. About 75% of sleep time is spent in this phase.

  $\mathcal{Q}$6. REM sleep is required for normal emotional functioning and is where we dream. It accounts for _____% of our sleep.

If you've been pulling an all-nighter to study for a pharmacology exam, more than the usual percentage of time will be spent in REM sleep the next time you snooze.

Sedatives and Hypnotics

Sedatives and hypnotics are used primarily to relieve anxiety and promote sleep. *Hypnotic* refers to the ability of a drug to induce sleep; **sedative** may not cause sleep, only relaxation. Whether a given drug causes sedation or sleep (hypnosis) is dose dependent.

Barbiturates

Barbiturates are powerful hypnotics. Almost all of them are metabolized in the liver. Duration of action ranges from 3 to 4 hours (secobarbital, pentobarbital) to 10 to 12 hours (phenobarbital). Repeated use or abuse of barbiturates leads to the development of tolerance, and increasing amounts of the drug are required to produce the desired effect. Elvis loved these!

Clinical Effects
The primary effect of barbiturates is the production of sedation, sleep, and anesthesia in a dose-dependent manner. Other clinical effects include the following:

- Respiratory depression—Barbiturates are used as a sleep aid. Be careful of the dose in patients with COPD or asthma.
- Cardiovascular depression—Use of barbiturates causes a drop in blood pressure, which is dose-dependent. There is greater sensitivity to cardiovascular effects in hypovolemia, CHF, or impaired cardiovascular function.

   Q 7. What clinical parameters should you monitor to assess cardiopulmonary status when giving barbiturates? _____

   _____

- Neuromuscular blockade—Use of barbiturates reduces the sensitivity of the postsynaptic membrane at the skeletal neuromuscular junction; the bottom line is muscle relaxation.
- Lack of analgesia—Sedation is not the same as analgesia. These are words to live by. Don't forget this when patients receiving ventilation are sedated. They may still be in pain.

Clinical Use of Barbiturates
- Sedation
- Anesthesia
- Sleep
- Anticonvulsant

Barbiturate Intoxication
Barbiturate intoxication is similar to having too much alcohol. It produces slurred speech, disorientation, and impaired motor skills.

   Q 8. Circle one. With severe intoxication, you see respiratory depression, which will cause respiratory (acidosis, alkalosis) and hypoxemia, coma, hypotension, cold clammy skin, and dilated pupils. What a pretty picture.

Treatment of barbiturate overdose includes the following:

- Ventilatory support
- Circulatory support
- Drug elimination
- Prevention of dehydration, infection, and other complications

Nonbarbiturate Sedatives and Hypnotics

Generally, nonbarbiturate sedatives and hypnotics are nonselective CNS depressants.

Benzodiazepine Hypnotics
Benzodiazepine hypnotics are widely used to relieve anxiety. They're minor tranquilizers.

Ethyl Alcohol
Don't forget the common drug ethyl alcohol. Alcohol has a depressant effect on the higher functions of the brain, including the RAS. Effects are proportional to the concentration of alcohol in the blood.

𝒬9. The first effects of alcohol are seen in loss of fine motor control and _____ reaction time. Enough ethyl alcohol (400 mg% or more) can dangerously depress the respiratory drive.

Effects
- Euphoria
- Cutaneous and peripheral vasodilation
- Diuresis

Alcohol has a positive interaction with sedatives, hypnotics, tranquilizers, and some analgesics.

Metabolism
Almost all ingested alcohol is oxidized to carbon dioxide and water. There are also some highly toxic intermediates formed.

𝒬10. Compare barbiturates and nonbarbiturates. Are the effects more similar or more different? _____
_____
_____
_____

Even though this has nothing to do with pharmacology per se, don't drink and drive or let your friends do so. A college friend of mine was killed by a drunk driver.

Anesthetics

General Anesthetics

Anesthesia means unconscious. This explains the whole section! General anesthesia (no relation to Captain Anesthesia of the Royal Canadian Mounties) causes CNS depression, producing total loss of consciousness and loss of reflexes. Following are the three types:

Barbiturate Anesthetics
Barbiturate anesthetics produce rapid and profound loss of consciousness, have a high lipid solubility, and quickly cross into the brain.

Their duration of action is short, and they produce no analgesia in a patient who's awake.

Nonbarbiturate Anesthetics
Nonbarbiturate anesthetics include a variety of drugs used for general anesthesia, twilight anesthesia, or conscious sedation during certain procedures. It's like you're not completely out or in.

Anesthetic Gases
Anesthetic gases are given with oxygen following induction of hypnosis using one of the agents we talked about earlier or after administration of a neuromuscular blocking agent before surgery. Anesthetic gases have a rapid onset of action.

𝒬11. Think of one *specific* situation where each of the three types of general anesthetics might be used.
1. _____
2. _____
3. _____

Local Anesthetics

The classic example of a local anesthetic is lidocaine. Another is procaine (Novocain).

Mechanism of Action
Remember, nerve impulses occur because of ion exchanges. A neuron is stimulated. Critical threshold is reached. Sodium channels open. Sodium flows in as a fast current to cause depolarization. Sodium channels close, and potassium channels open.

Well, local anesthetics bind to sodium channels, blocking the inward sodium current. This increases the critical threshold. Impulse conduction is slowed. The nerve is no longer able to generate an action potential in response to a stimulus. There's no sedation, you just can't feel the pain of the dentist's drill!

Psychotherapeutic Agents

Minor Tranquilizers

Minor tranquilizers belong to the benzodiazepine group. A classic example is diazepam (Valium). (Remember the Rolling Stones' "Mother's Little Helper"?) The minor tranquilizers have the following advantages over the barbiturates:

- No respiratory depression at sedative doses
- High TI

Do you remember what a high TI is? Define it here. _____
_____

Answer: In case you were too lazy to look back in the book, it means there's a big difference between the lethal and therapeutic doses of the drug (always nice).

Tranquilizers are used to treat neuroses and anxiety. Midazolam (Versed) is another commonly used example. Flumazenil can be given to reverse the effects of benzodiazepines, which is awfully nice.

Antipsychotic Drugs (Neuroleptics)

Antipsychotic drugs are used to alleviate the symptoms of more severe mental illness, like schizophrenia, mania, and organic brain syndrome. They are also sometimes used to treat manic-depression. These agents aren't curative, but they do alleviate the symptoms. Basically, neuroleptic drugs act by blocking dopamine receptor sites in the limbic system.

Side Effects
Antipsychotic drugs block cholinergic receptors, so they produce the following:

- Tachycardia
- Dry mouth
- Blurred vision
- Urinary retention
- Constipation
- Decreased respiratory secretions

Some effects are dose related. Their effects on the cerebral cortex include sedation and ataxia.

_Q_12. At high doses, antipsychotic drugs suppress respiration and may cause cardiovascular collapse, which may result in
_____.

Cholinesterase Inhibitors

Used to treat Alzheimer's disease, cholinesterase inhibitors slow the progress but do not stop the disease process.

_Q_13. Cholinergic neurotransmission in the lung can cause bronchoconstriction, so carefully monitor the use of cholinesterase inhibitors in patients with _____ and _____.

Lithium

Lithium is used to treat manic-depression. Lithium decreases the pressor response to norepinephrine, so it should be used with caution in patients with compromised cardiovascular function.

Antidepressants

There are two types of depression:

1. Reactive—related to a traumatic life event

2. Endogenous depression—caused by a neurotransmitter imbalance in the limbic system, involving norepinephrine and serotonin. There are three types of antidepressants—tricyclics, tetracyclics, and monamine oxidase-inhibitors (MAOIs). All three types increase norepinephrine and serotonin.

Tricyclics and Tetracyclics

Tricyclics and tetracyclics produce cholinergic receptor blockade peripherally. Anticholinergic side effects are the same as with the neuroleptics.

Q 14. List the anticholinergic side effects caused by neuroleptics, tricyclics, and tetracyclics.

_____

_____

The primary CNS side effect is sedation. Toxic doses cause a generalized CNS stimulation, followed by CNS depression.

Monoamine Oxidase Inhibitors

Q 15. MAO is an _____ (*ase* always indicates an enzyme) found in the gastrointestinal tract, liver, and nerve endings that uses norepinephrine as its neurotrasmitter. MAOIs increase the concentration of epinephrine, norepinephrine, and serotonin. This causes the antidepressant effect.

Q 16. MAO toxicity causes CNS stimulation, then depression, similar to the _____. Hypertensive crisis is a serious side effect of MAOIs. Monitor the respiratory and cardiovascular systems closely.

Analgesics

There are two types of analgesics—narcotics and nonnarcotics.

NARCOTICS

Derived from opium, narcotic analgesics produce their therapeutic effect by combining with specific receptor sites found throughout the nervous system such as subcortical regions of the brain and in the spinal cord. Opioids inhibit the release of excitatory transmitters, blocking the transmission of pain perception.

Pharmacological Properties of Morphine

The effects of morphine and its derivatives are listed below.

- Analgesia
- Euphoria
- Sedation
- Respiratory depression
- Cough suppression
- Miosis
- Trunk rigidity
- Nausea/vomiting
- Constipation

Q 17. With depression of the respiratory center, the response to high carbon dioxide levels is _____.

Q 18. What effect on respiration would a huge dose of morphine have?

_____

_____

Opioids also produce constricted pupils. The classic pinpoint pupil is a tell-tale sign of opioid overdose.

Morphine-induced release of histamine can cause increased airway resistance/bronchospasm.

Q 19. So the use of narcotics is discouraged in which patient population?

_____

As with many of the drugs we've covered in this chapter, there is potential for abuse and addiction with opioids.

Therapeutic Use of Narcotics
- Pain relief
- Cough suppression
- Relief of dyspnea caused by left ventricular failure
- Sedation
- Antidiarrhea

Narcotics decrease peripheral vascular resistance and increase venous reservoir to reduce the work of the left ventricle.

Overdose of Morphine and Its Derivatives

Opioid overdose is characterized by pinpoint pupils, coma, and depressed ventilation. In barbiturate overdose, the pupils are dilated, so it's usually easy to distinguish the two. The therapeutic dose of morphine is 10 mg IM or subcutaneous in the adult. Doses higher than 100 mg may be fatal; 300 mg is considered lethal. Addicts can tolerate up to 5 g/day. Yikes!

Q 20. How many milligrams is 5 g? _____

IV overdose of heroin may result in pulmonary edema, ARDS, hypoxia, and pulmonary exudate.

Examples of opioid analgesics include morphine, opium, and codeine.

Narcotic Antagonists

There are drugs (naloxone [Narcan] and Naltrexone) that can cancel the effects of narcotics. They're pure antagonists, so if you give it to someone who's addicted to one of the narcotics, they'll experience an immediate withdrawal symptom. If a mother is given narcotics to treat the delivery process pain, naloxone is used in the neonate to reverse depressed ventilation. I'll bet lots of neonates get this. I know I was screaming for drugs! Thanks for sharing.

If you're using naloxone to reverse narcotic overdose, you've got to give repeated doses because it's metabolized rapidly.

Nonnarcotic Analgesics

Nonnarcotic drugs are used to reduce elevated body temperature and to promote analgesia. Examples of these agents are salicylates (aspirin), aniline derivatives (acetaminophen), and nonsteroidal antiinflammatory drugs, or NSAID (ibuprofen).

Salicylates

Effects include analgesia, antipyresis, and antiinflammation. Salicylates also inhibit hemostasis (a not-so-hot effect) through platelet inhibition. When absorbed from the stomach, aspirin and other salicylates can cause ulceration of gastric mucosa and gastric bleeding.

In what patient populations would salicylates be contraindicated?

_____

_____

Answer: Salicylates should not be given to patients with hemophilia, or those receiving anticoagulant therapy.

Aspirin overdose leads to metabolic acidosis. When your carbon dioxide level is high, what does your body do to compensate?

_____

Answer: Your body hyperventilates.

This is why victims of aspirin overdose exhibit Kussmaul breathing (increased rate and depth).

Because of its antiinflammatory effect, salicylates are used in the treatment of rheumatoid arthritis. In certain asthmatic patients, salicylates have caused bronchospasm.

Q 21. List at least two patient populations who would probably benefit from aspirin.
    1. _____
    2. _____
    3. Only overachievers complete this line.
      _____

Q 22. List three populations who would probably not benefit from aspirin treatment.
    1. _____
    2. _____
    3. _____

Aniline Derivatives

Examples of aniline derivatives are acetaminophen and phenacetin. They have both the analgesic and antipyretic effects of aspirin but none of the nasty side effects, like clotting interference.

The bad news is that acetaminophen overdose causes hepatotoxicity.

*Q*23. Remember what the treatment for acetaminophen overdose is? (hint: a mucolytic?)

_____

*Q*24. Review the mechanism by which acetylcysteine can save the liver and write it here:

_____

_____

_____

Aniline derivatives are good alternative analgesics for people with hemophilia, aspirin sensitivity combined with asthma, or ulcers.

Nonsteroidal Antiinflammatory Drugs
Nonsteroidal antinflammatory drugs (NSAIDs) were the result of the search for a less toxic antiinflammatory with fewer side effects. NSAIDs have analgesic, antipyretic, and antiinflammatory effects. They are used to treat: the following:

• Rheumatoid arthritis
• Osteoarthritis
• Mild to moderate pain associated with dental work or soft tissue injuries
• Primary dysmenorrhea
• Sunburn
• Prevention of migraine headaches

NSAIDs inhibit prostaglandin and leukotriene synthesis, so asthmatic individuals may also be sensitive to this group of drugs.

*Q*25. How are NSAIDs similar to aniline derivatives? _____

_____

*Q*26. How are NSAIDs similar to aspirin?

_____

_____

Respiratory Stimulants

Respiratory stimulants are CNS stimulants that increase rather than depress the respiratory drive. Because the CNS is stimulated, central respiratory centers in the medulla are also stimulated. A respiratory stimulant should selectively affect only the respiratory center, but the analeptics in use are all general stimulants. The adverse effects are a result of this nonspecificity and include the following:

• Restlessness   • Sweating
• Hypertension   • Tachycardia
• Vomiting   • Hyperpyrexia

Greater stimulation can cause convulsions.

Agents

Analeptics, like doxapram, are the safest. Doxapram more selectively stimulates the peripheral chemoreceptors. It's usually given IV, with ventilatory effects seldom lasting longer than 5 to 10 minutes with a bolus dose. Longterm effects require continuous infusion, which increases the risk of side effects.

Remember the xanthines, often used as bronchodilators? They're also respiratory stimulants.

The salicylates (aspirin) are also capable of stimulating ventilation (remember Kussmaul breathing).

*Q*27. Take a look back at the analgesic section, review the mechanism, and explain in your own words how aspirin could be a respiratory stimulant. _____

_____

_____

_____

Progesterone, an ovarian hormone, has been noted to stimulate ventilation with parenteral administration. Go figure!

Clinical Use

CNS stimulants are limited in a bizillion ways. Listed below are some cases where you might think they should be used, along with the reason why CNS stimulants are a bad idea!

1. Sedative-Hypnotic Overdose

Ventilatory support is much easier and safer.

2. Chronic Ventilatory Failure

Analeptics don't do any good for chronic problems because their effect is transitory.

3. Acute Ventilatory Failure

Why try to stimulate a pulmonary system that's already incapable of continuing the work of breathing? It's like beating a dead horse.

4. Acute-on-Chronic Ventilatory Failure

An analeptic increases the work of breathing and oxygen consumption, haven't you been listening?

5. Postanesthesia Recovery

Temporary ventilatory support is safer than using analeptics.

*Q*28. Reversal of narcotics with _____ is a better idea.

6. Miscellaneous Application

Here are the only places where doxapram and other analeptics have been used with some success:

- To reverse hypercapnia and hypoventilation in perinatal respiratory depression
- Congenital central hypoventilation syndromes
- Obesity-hypoventilation syndromes

These are the final 10 NBRC questions. I'll give you a minute to wipe the tear from your eye.

1. Which of the following CNS structures is responsible for controlling blood pressure and ventilation?
   a. Cerebral cortex
   b. Midbrain
   c. Medulla
   d. Hypothalamus   (Chapter 22, p. 342)

2. Drugs that affect CNS function:
   I.   Do so in a descending fashion
   II. Do so in an ascending fashion
   III. Do not appear to be dose related
   IV. Are dose related

   a. I and III
   b. I and IV
   c. II and III
   d. II and IV   (Chapter 22, p. 343)

3. All but which of the following are true of REM sleep?
   a. We spend 75% of our sleep in this state.
   b. We dream here.
   c. We need it for normal emotional functioning.
   d. Sleep deprivation is "made up" in the REM state.   (Chapter 22, p. 343)

4. Barbiturates are classified as which of the following?
   a. Local anesthetics
   b. Hypnotics
   c. Narcotics
   d. Antipsychotics   (Chapter 22, p. 344)

5. All but which of the following are true of ethyl alcohol?
   a. It is a CNS depressant.
   b. It has a positive interaction with sedatives.
   c. It is oxidized to carbon dioxide and water.
   d. It stimulates the respiratory drive.
                         (Chapter 22, p. 348)

6. Which of the following describes anesthetic gases?
   a. Have a rapid onset of action
   b. Are administered prior to the induction of hypnosis
   c. Can be addictive
   d. b and c   (Chapter 22, pp. 349-350)

7. Compared to barbiturates, minor tranquilizers accomplish which of the following?
   a. Have a lower therapeutic index
   b. Affect sodium influx
   c. Do not depress the respiratory drive
   d. a and c   (Chapter 22, p. 351)

8. Which of the following applies to narcotic analgesics?
   a. Block the transmission of pain perception
   b. Can depress the medullary respiratory center
   c. Are potentially addictive
   d. All the above(Chapter 22, pp. 354-355)

9. All but which of the following are considered to be therapeutic uses for narcotics?
   a. Expectorant
   b. Pain relief
   c. Sedation
   d. Relief of dyspnea caused by left ventricular failure
                       (Chapter 22, pp. 355-356)

10. Which of the following statements are true of naloxone (Narcan)?
    I.   It is classified as a narcotic antagonist.
    II. It is used in certain neonates.
    III. It metabolizes slowly.
    IV. It contributes to respiratory depression.

    a. I, II, III
    b. II, III, IV
    c. II and IV
    d. I and II   (Chapter 22, p. 357)

Sim
There is a new resident at your hospital, who is a big fan of doxapram. What is doxapram?

_____

_____

Answer: It's an analeptic respiratory stimulant. Effects on ventilation last about 5 to 10 minutes.

The resident is dying to use it on a patient. (I guess she doesn't get out much.) Anyway, she pages you about every 30 minutes with a new patient who would benefit from it. How will you thwart her enthusiasm with each of the scenarios?

1. A 67-year-old COPD patient has been admitted with pneumonia.

   _____
   _____
   _____

Answer: This represents acute-on-chronic respiratory failure. It won't work because doxapram's effects are transitory, the work of breathing will be increased and so will oxygen consumption.

2. A 32-year-old patient is status-post wedge resection (part of his/her lung has been removed) and deteriorating (ventilatory-wise) in the recovery room. Wouldn't a little respiratory stimulant do wonders? _____

   _____
   _____

Answer: Temporary ventilatory support is safer than using doxapram.

3. What if another recovery room patient got a little too much narcotic anesthetic and is having some trouble coming around. Breathing is a little shallow. Doxapram to the rescue? Intubation?

   _____
   _____
   _____

Answer: Administer naloxone (Narcan)!

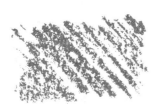

Answer Key

Chapter 1

Q 1. drugs—cardiopulmonary disease—critical care

Q 2. toxicology

Q 3. c

Q 4. d

Q 5. a

Q 6. 2—4—3—1

Q 7. Advantage—It's good that there's a drug available to treat rare diseases; Disadvantage—It's expensive to develop and market the drug.

Q 8. False

Q 9. False

Q10. Any OTC drug could be listed. Examples are aspirin, cough and cold medicines, Benadryl, Primatene Mist, etc.

Q11. 1—G
2—D
3—E
4—F
5—C
6—B
7—A

Q12. antiinfective

Q13. antiarrhythmic

NBRC Questions

1. d
2. b
3. d
4. b
5. a

Chapter 2

Q 1. False

Q 2. either

Q 3. systemic

Q 4. either

Q 5. either

Q 6. nonionized, lipid-soluble

Q 7. aqueous is passive; facilitated is active

Q 8. Dose = V_D × Concentration
100 mg = V_D × 5 mg/L
V_D = 100/5 = 20

Q 9. decreases

Q10. salmeterol

Q11. long-lasting, slow to peak, lasts overnight

Q12. isoetharine

Q13. quick peak effect, doesn't last long

Q14. fewer systemic side effects

Q15. 90%

Q16. 10%

Q17. 1:2

Q18. fewer

Q19. nonionized

Q20. G—adenylyl cyclase—transmembrane signaling

Q21. drug B

Q22. dangerous

Q23. less efficacy

Q24. Agonist

Q25. Antagonist

Q26. idiosyncratic

NBRC Questions

1. a
2. b
3. a
4. d
5. c
6. b
7. b
8. a
9. c
10. d

Chapter 3

Q 1. stability—penetration

Q 2. Advantages—smaller doses, quick action, acts directly on the respiratory system, fewer side effects, convenient, painless; Disadvantages—many factors affect penetration, difficult to calculate correct dose and replicate it, MDI use may be difficult for some patients

Q 3. The goal of aerosol therapy is penetration into the lower respiratory tract. The greater the number of properly sized aerosol particles (1 to 5 μm), the greater the number that reach the lower respiratory tract.

Q 4. While sitting up, take slow deep breaths and try to hold your breath about every fifth breath; breath through your mouth

Q 5. 1 to 5 μm

Q 6. SVN advantage—cheaper, do not need an electrical source; USN advantage—faster treatment time, do not need a gas source, produces an aerosol that is more dense

Q 7. Filling volume—3 to 4 ml; Treatment time—about 10 minutes; Flow rate—6 to 8 L/min

Q 8. Put the canister into the actuator connector. Press down on it. Drug and propellant mix and get released. Mixture vaporizes when it hits the air. An aerosol is created.

Q 9. Gather supplies. Assemble inhaler. (Remove cap!) If you don't have a spacer, hold the MDI an inch away from your mouth. Exhale normally. Begin taking a deep breath slowly. Press down on the canister as you are inhaling. Hold your breath as long as you can (up to 10 seconds). Wait 30 seconds between puffs. Replace cap.

Q 10. Reservoirs have one-way valves, spacers don't.

Q 11. No CFC propellants, easy to tell how much drug is left (count the capsules).

NBRC Questions

1. c
2. a
3. d
4. a
5. d
6. b
7. d
8. c
9. d
10. a

Chapter 4

Q 1. 510
Q 2. 33,000
Q 3. 0.024
Q 4. 1700
Q 5. 68,000,000—68,000
Q 6. 48
Q 7. 8
Q 8. 0.125
Q 9. 0.000003

1. c
2. b
3. d
4. a
5. a
6. c
7. c
8. c
9. b
10. b

Chapter 5

Q 1. if you've got to get out of a burning building; if a bully is chasing you for your lunch money—you get the idea

Q 2. 1—E
2—H
3—G
4—D
5—C
6—B
7—F
8—A

Q 3. both alpha and beta

Q 4. vagus—muscarinic—airway smooth—bronchoconstriction—submucosal glands—cholinesterase

NBRC Questions

1. d
2. b
3. c
4. a
5. b
6. c
7. d
8. a
9. c
10. c

Chapter 6

Q 1. salmeterol

Q 2. vasoconstriction, decongestion

Q 3. increased heart rate and force of contraction

Q 4. bronchodilation, inhibition of inflammation, increased mucociliary clearance

Q 5. works fast, doesn't last long

Q 6. short—COMT

Q 7. liver—gut

Q 8. lasts longer, slower to peak, not inactivated by COMT (these make saligenins good for maintenance); beta-2 specific

Q 9. very beta-2 specific

*Q*10. Maintenance drugs would be of little or no benefit to the person having an asthma attack because they are slow to peak.

*Q*11. catecholamines—derivatives of catecholamines

*Q*12. COMT—oral

*Q*13. spacer/reservoir

*Q*14. fewer

*Q*15. inhaled

*Q*16. cardiac

*Q*17. should *never*

*Q*18. corticosteroids

NBRC Questions

1. c
2. a
3. b
4. d
5. c
6. b
7. d
8. b
9. d
10. d
11. d

Chapter 7

Q 1. blocking the action of acetylcholine; acetylcholine causes bronchoconstriction

Q 2. indirectly

Q 3. tertiary ammonium compounds

Q 4. ipratropium bromide—lesser

Q 5. tertiary ammonium

Q 6. increase—increase

Q 7. quaternary ammonium

Q 8. MDI—32 μg; SVN—500 μg

Q 9. SVN; more drug equals more side effects

Q 10. bronchodilation—bronchoconstriction

Q 11. albuterol—ipratropium—more

NBRC Questions

1. c
2. d
3. a
4. c
5. b
6. d
7. b
8. d
9. c
10. c

Chapter 8

Q 1. Caffeine—to stay awake; Theophylline—to treat bronchoconstriction

Q 2. 2— 1—3

Q 3. 3—1—2

Q 4. 5 to 15 μg/ml

Q 5. 10 to 12 μg/ml

Q 6. The drug will have no therapeutic effect.

Q 7. Increase the dose.

Q 8. 400 mg/day

Q 9. Decrease the dose and check a blood level.

Q 10. 10 to 20 μg/ml

Q 11. Drink lots of water (at least 8 glasses/day, more with exercise); limit caffeine intake (coffee, tea, soda).

Q 12. nausea, vomiting, abdominal pain, supraventricular tachycardia, increased respiratory rate, palpitations, ventricular dysrhythmias, diuresis, headache, anxiety, tremor, convulsions

NBRC Questions

1. c
2. b
3. a
4. b
5. b
6. d
7. a
8. c
9. c
10. a

Chapter 9

Q 1. 5

Q 2. 6800 × 5 = 34,000

Q 3. 1—E
2—D
3—F
4—B
5—C
6—A

Q 4. A 60-year-old COPD patient who smokes, lives in Los Angeles, has a trach, is hypoxemic, takes ipratropium bromide (Atrovent) and cough syrup with codeine, who will be given general anesthesia for _____ (pick a surgery).

Q 5. ciliary beat, mucus production, mucus transport

Q 6. mucus production

Q 7.

Q 8. It's hard to get rid of it. Patients may get bacterial infection. Mucus thickens. Ciliary beat slows or stops, which leads to airway obstruction. Atelectasis may result.

Q 9. tomato sauce

Q 10. rubber band

Q 11. 10 or 20%

Q 12. It will take the appropriate time to nebulize (about 10 minutes).

Q 13. asthma

Q 14. isoetharine; metaproterenol

Q 15. antibiotics

Q 16. acetaminophen

Q 17. Acetylcysteine neutralizes the toxic metabolite, protecting the liver from destruction.

Q 18. thickness

Q 19. Thinner mucus is easier to get rid of.

Q 20. viscous

NBRC Questions

1. a
2. c
3. b
4. b
5. c
6. a
7. c
8. b
9. d
10. c

Chapter 10

Q 1. lower—force—alveolus—easier

Q 2. from humans, from animals, from synthetic material

Q 3. high

Q 4. lamellar bodies—alveolus

Q 5. type II—secreted

Q 6. Natural surfactant:
Advantage—has all the right ingredients already
Disadvantage—expensive and hard to get
Synthetic surfactant:
Advantage—no contamination
Disadvantage—doesn't work as well as natural surfactant does

Q 7. There's not enough of it.

Q 8. If the lungs are able to stay inflated, there's more room for gas exchange.

Q 9. Exosurf—synthetic; dose is 5 ml/kg; must be reconstituted; if more than one dose is required, it's given every 12 hours; administered through the endotracheal tube via a side port; baby gets half the dose on the right side, is turned, and receives the remaining half on the left side. Survanta—modified natural surfactant; doesn't have to be reconstituted; delivered through a catheter in the endotracheal tube

NBRC Questions

1. d
2. b
3. b
4. c
5. d
6. c
7. d
8. d
9. b
10. b

Chapter 11

Q 1. outer zone

Q 2. When your body produces its own glucocorticoids, a feedback mechanism in your body limits their production. The same thing happens when you give exogenous corticosteroids.

Q 3. Adrenal suppression would occur both in the morning (naturally) and at bedtime. Every day administration would also result in excessive adrenal suppression.

Q 4. decreased/minimized

Q 5. decreased mucus secretion; decreased plasma leakage; restored responsiveness to beta agonists

Q 6. Flovent

Q 7. It's given bid versus tid or qid for Decadron.

Q 8. It's a controller, not a reliever.

Q 9. decreased systemic side effects; decreased amount of drug deposited in the oropharynx

Q 10. parasympatholytic (anticholinergic)

NBRC Questions
1. b
2. a
3. c
4. c
5. a
6. c
7. b
8. c
9. d
10. d

Chapter 12

Q 1. decreased

Q 2. Extrinsic—caused by an allergy, more common in kids; Intrinsic—not associated with allergens, more common in adults

Q 3. 1. bronchoconstriction
2. mucosal edema
3. secretion of mucous
4. cytokines or eosinophils

Q 4. sympathomimetic (adrenergic), parasympatholytic (anticholinergic), xanthines

Q 5. bronchoconstriction, mucosal edema, increased secretions

Q 6. d

Q 7. osteoporosis plus the other nasty side effects, like Cushing's syndrome, etc.

Q 8. an acute asthma attack

Q 9. If patients can take their medicine less often, they're usually more compliant.

Q 10. controller—an acute asthma attack

Q 11. Zafirlukast—use in those older than 12 years, available in tablet form or inhaled, acts on leukotrienes, works on intrinsic asthma
Zileuton—use on those older than 12 years, works on leukotrienes, available in tablet form, may affect liver function

NBRC Questions
1. b
2. d
3. c
4. b
5. d
6. a
7. c
8. a
9. c
10. d

Chapter 13

Q 1. Pentamidine isethionate binds to tissue in the major organs and may remain there for up to 9 months.

Q 2. hypoglycemia and impaired renal function

Q 3. Administer a bronchodilator with aerosolized pentamidine, probably a fast-acting sympathomimetic.

Q 4. 1, 2, 3, 4, 6, 7, 8

Q 5. 5

Q 6. prevent viral entry into the cell; prevent viral replication; prevent viral exit from the cell

Q 7. younger than 2 years with a history of bronchopulmonary dysplasia; younger than 2 years with a history of premature birth

Q 8. intravenous administration

Q 9. 10 to12 L/min

Q 10. same as anything else, 6 to 8 L/min

Q 11. bronchodilator

NBRC Questions
1. c
2. d
3. b
4. d
5. b
6. b
7. d
8. a
9. b
10. c

Chapter 14

Q 1. *Antiinfective* is a broader term. It includes drugs toxic to bacteria and many other microorganisms.

Q 2. *Staphylococcus aureus* can produce an enzyme (penicillinase or beta-lactamase) that can actually inactivate certain antibiotics. Feel free to choose any of the bacteria listed in 1 through 4 on p. 00 and describe their defense mechanism.

Q 3. *Streptococcus pneumoniae*

Q 4. Penicillinase is an enzyme that inactivates penicillin.

Q 5. penicillins

Q 6. screwing up bacterial wall synthesis

Q 7. carbapenems, cephalosporins, penicillins

Q 8. monbactam, carbapenems, cephalosporins

Q 9. kidney (renal)—liver (hepatic)

Q 10. people with renal failure, people with hepatic dysfunction, kids

Q 11. aminoglycosides

Q 12. streptomycin

Q 13. tetracycline

Q 14. cephalosporin

Q 15. cephalosporin

Q 16. erythromycin

Q 17. Use a spacer. Rinse mouth after use.

Q 18. Multiple drugs are used and must be taken for so long that patients may not be compliant with therapy.

Q 19. False

Q 20. False

NBRC Questions
1. c
2. a
3. b
4. c
5. d
6. c
7. b
8. a
9. d
10. d

Chapter 15

Q 1. increased heart rate—strength of contraction

Q 2. bronchoconstriction, skin reactions, mucus secretion, and nasal congestion

Q 3. impacted secretions

Q 4. swollen mucosa, tolerance

Q 5. upper airway drying, sedative effect

Q 6. may be increased secretion production (with certain types), which is a real problem if the patient cannot clear the secretions

Q 7. not good for patients who need to clear secretions (cystic fibrosis, COPD, chronic bronchitis)

NBRC Questions

1. a
2. b
3. b
4. d
5. b
6. d
7. d
8. c
9. c
10. d

Chapter 16

 1. Elastase is an enzyme in your lung that eats alveolar tissue. Alpha-1 antitrypsin holds it in check. If you don't have enough alpha-1 antitrypsin, your alveolar walls are systematically destroyed, resulting in emphysema.

 2. 60 mg/kg × 50 kg = 3000 mg

 3. yes or no (Don't you love these?!)

 4. irritable, anxious, unable to concentrate, gaining weight (need to have something in the mouth all the time), nicotine craving . . .

 5. smokes more than 15 cigarettes per day with frequent, deep inhalations; smokes a cigarette first thing in the morning; smokes more in the morning than in the evening

 6. Nicotine gum—Advantage: absorption of nicotine is fast; Disadvantage: it tastes bad and may make you nauseous
Nicotine patch—Advantage: available in various strengths; Disadvantage: skin irritation
Nicotine nasal spray—Advantage: rapid peak plasma levels of nicotine; Disadvantage: may cause runny nose, watery eyes

 7. smoke

 8. buildup of nicotine—cardiac dysrhythmias

 9. no, only pulmonary vasodilation

10. Nitric oxide decreases PVR.

11. Nitric oxide may cause pulmonary edema.

NBRC Questions

1. b
2. d
3. c
4. b
5. d
6. a
7. c
8. d
9. c
10. b

Chapter 17

 1. neonate and swallowing a pill; infant and MDI or DPI

 2. topical, IV, IM

 3. water-soluble

 4. impairs/hampers

 5. Young's rule: $\frac{10}{10+12} \times 10$ mg
= 10/22 × 10 mg
= 0.45 × 10 = 4.5 mg
(In reality, the adult and children's doses are equal.)

 6. 10%

 7. They cannot generate flow rates higher than 60 L/min.

NBRC Questions

1. b
2. a
3. c
4. b
5. d
6. d
7. d
8. a
9. d
10. b

Chapter 18

Q 1. small

Q 2. biceps, triceps, quadriceps, diaphragm, hamstrings . . .

Q 3. Depolarization—Muscle is permeable to sodium ions. Critical threshold is reached. Muscle reaches its action potential. Cells release calcium ions. Muscle contraction occurs.
Repolarization—Membrane potential returns to normal. Sodium conduction is blocked. Sodium-potassium exchange occurs. The muscle is ready for depolarization (contraction) again.

Q 4. rapid

Q 5. breathing

Q 6. vision

Q 7. The patient may have difficulty breathing. This is never good.

Q 8. asthmatic patients

Q 9. If muscles (any muscle, even those used to breathe) aren't used, they become less efficient. Thus weaning will be harder and take longer because the muscles are weak. It's like when you first start lifting weights, you've got to build up the muscle before you can lift like Arnold!

*Q*10. asthmatic patients

*Q*11. IV

*Q*12. paralysis

*Q*13. decrease

NBRC Questions

1. a
2. d
3. b
4. d
5. a
6. d
7. c
8. c
9. b
10. b

Chapter 19

Q 1. decrease—increase

Q 2. increase

Q 3. decrease

Q 4. increase

Q 5. Increased preload (volume) will increase cardiac output to a point. If the volume becomes overwhelming for the heart to handle, cardiac output will decrease.

Q 6. inotropic

Q 7. digoxin

Q 8. right ventricular preload, filling pressure

Q 9. increase—decrease

*Q*10. PAWP will decrease.

*Q*11. increasing

*Q*12. bronchodilation

*Q*13. heart rate—strength of contraction

*Q*14. strength of contraction

*Q*15. increase

*Q*16. Action potential—depolarization and repolarization of the heart

*Q*17. 1. propranolol—beta-adrenergic blocker—slows supraventricular tachycardia
2. verapamil—calcium channel blocker—supraventricular tachycardia
3. quinidine—membrane stabilizer—atrial and ventricular dysrhythmias
4. lidocaine—membrane stabilizer—PVCs, ventricular tachycardia, ventricular fibrillation

*Q*18. EMD—electrical activity without pumping blood

NBRC Questions
1. c
2. a
3. d
4. a
5. d
6. c
7. c
8. b
9. c
10. b

NBRC Questions
1. b
2. c
3. d
4. c
5. d
6. a
7. c
8. b
9. d
10. d

Chapter 20

𝒬 1. decreased

𝒬 2. decreased

𝒬 3. heart

𝒬 4. alpha—beta

𝒬 5. decreases

𝒬 6. Angina increases oxygen demand on the heart.

𝒬 7. antiarrhythmic

𝒬 8. 1

𝒬 9. Nitrates and nitrites—yes—no
Calcium channel blockers—yes—no
Beta-adrenergic blockers—yes—no

𝒬10. a blood clot that obstructs a vessel or cavity of the heart

𝒬11. Heparin binds to this anticlot substance, which won't allow fibrinogen to change into fibrin. Fibrin is what forms a clot.

𝒬12. Difference—Heparin is used for acute care treatment; coumarin is used for long-term treatment.
Similarity—The effect of either heparin or warfarin should be monitored via blood tests.

Chapter 21

𝒬 1. an active organ

𝒬 2. low chloride—low potassium

𝒬 3. decrease

𝒬 4. neither

𝒬 5. metabolic acidosis

𝒬 6. metabolic alkalosis

𝒬 7. metabolic alkalosis

NBRC Questions
1. d
2. d
3. a
4. c
5. b
6. c
7. a
8. d
9. b
10. d

Chapter 22

𝒬 1. increased ventilation

𝒬 2. ventilation

𝒬 3. slows

𝒬 4. decreases

𝒬 5. cortex—depressing—death

𝒬 6. 25

Q 7. blood pressure; respiratory rate (heart rate wouldn't hurt.)

Q 8. acidosis

Q 9. decreased/slowed

Q 10. more similar

Q 11. 1. intubating a trauma victim
2. dental procedures, like a root canal
3. open heart surgery

Q 12. death

Q 13. asthma—COPD

Q 14. tachycardia, dry mouth, constipation, blurred vision, decreased respiratory secretions, urinary retention

Q 15. enzyme

Q 16. tricyclics

Q 17. hyperventilation

Q 18. depression of the respiratory drive

Q 19. asthmatic patients

Q 20. 5000 mg

Q 21. 1. patients with rheumatoid arthritis
2. patients whose blood is "thick" (like patients with COPD and polycythemia)
3. patients in pain who cannot tolerate NSAIDs.

Q 22. 1. patients with hemophilia
2. patients with ulcers
3. patients taking anticoagulants

Q 23. acetylcysteine (Mucomyst)

Q 24. Acetylcysteine binds the toxic metabolite that destroys the liver.

Q 25. antipyretic, no clotting interference

Q 26. Asthmatic individuals may be sensitive to NSAIDs and aspirin.

Q 27. Aspirin overdose leads to metabolic acidosis, increased $PaCO_2$ levels, and hyperventilation

Q 28. naloxone (Narcan)

NBRC Questions
1. c
2. b
3. a
4. b
5. d
6. a
7. c
8. d
9. a
10. d